P9-DDK-659

I'VE GOT
YOUR BACK

I'VE GOT YOUR BACK

THE TRUTH ABOUT BACK SURGERY, STRAIGHT FROM A SURGEON

Nathaniel L. Tindel, MD, with
Tamar Haspel

New American Library

New American Library
Published by New American Library, a division of Penguin Group (USA) Inc., 375 Hudson Street,
New York, New York 10014, USA
Penguin Group (Canada), 90 Eglinton Avenue East, Suite 700, Toronto,
Ontario M4P 2Y3, Canada (a division of Pearson Penguin Canada Inc.)
Penguin Books Ltd., 80 Strand, London WC2R 0RL, England
Penguin Ireland, 25 St. Stephen's Green, Dublin 2,
Ireland (a division of Penguin Books Ltd.)
Penguin Group (Australia), 250 Camberwell Road, Camberwell, Victoria 3124,
Australia (a division of Pearson Australia Group Pty. Ltd.)
Penguin Books India Pvt. Ltd., 11 Community Centre, Panchsheel Park,
New Delhi - 110 017, India
Penguin Group (NZ), cnr Airborne and Rosedale Roads, Albany,
Auckland 1310, New Zealand (a division of Pearson New Zealand Ltd.)
Penguin Books (South Africa) (Pty.) Ltd., 24 Sturdee Avenue,
Rosebank, Johannesburg 2196, South Africa

Penguin Books Ltd., Registered Offices: 80 Strand, London WC2R 0RL, England

First published by New American Library, a division of Penguin Group (USA) Inc.

First Printing, January 2007
10 9 8 7 6 5 4 3 2 1

Copyright © Nathaniel L. Tindel, MD, and Tamar Haspel, 2007
Illustrations by Andrew Evansen
All rights reserved

REGISTERED TRADEMARK—MARCA REGISTRADA

LIBRARY OF CONGRESS CATALOGING-IN-PUBLICATION DATA

Tindel, Nathaniel L.
  I've got your back: the truth about back surgery, straight from a surgeon/Nathaniel L. Tindel with Tamar
Haspel.
    p. cm.
  ISBN-13: 978-0-451-22021-9
  1. Back—Surgery—Popular works.   I. Haspel, Tamar.   II. Title.
RD768.T56 2007
617.5'6059—dc22   2006028535

Set in Sabon & Frutiger
Designed by BTD NYC

Printed in the United States of America

PUBLISHER'S NOTE
The case studies in this book are based on real patients and events. The names and circumstances of all of them
have been changed to protect their identities.
    Every effort as been made to ensure that the information contained in this book is complete and accurate.
However, neither the publisher nor the authors are engaged in rendering professional advice or services to the
individual reader. The ideas, procedures, and suggestions contained in this book are not intended as a substitute
for consulting with your physician. All matters regarding your health require medical supervision. Neither the authors nor the publisher shall be liable or responsible for any loss or damage allegedly arising from any information or suggestion in this book. The opinions expressed in this book represent the personal views of the authors
and not of the publisher.
    While the authors have made every effort to provide accurate telephone numbers and Internet addresses at
the time of publication, neither the publisher nor the authors assume any responsibility for errors, or for changes
that occur after publication. Further, the publisher does not have any control over and does not assume any responsibility for author or third-party Web sites or their content.

TO THE MEMORY OF
MY FATHER AND BEST FRIEND,
Seymour Tindel, MD

ACKNOWLEDGMENTS

I could not have written this book if it weren't for all of my patients, colleagues, teachers, residents-in-training, and students who continue to challenge me when it comes to the complex world of back pain.

I would like to specifically recognize my spine fellowship mentors: Frank J. Eismont, MD, Nathan H. Lebwohl, MD, Mark D. Brown, MD, and Harry Shufflebarger, MD, for teaching me the foundations that I rely on when I treat patients with difficult spine problems.

I am grateful to my preceptor at Princeton University, Malcolm S. Steinberg, for allowing me to explore my scientific pursuits as an undergraduate. I would also like to thank R. Bruce Heppenstall, MD, my mentor in medical school at The University of Pennsylvania School of Medicine, who convinced me to become an orthopaedic surgeon instead of a cardiovascular surgeon. I was fortunate to spend time and gain valuable experience with some of the greatest physicians I know at Boston Children's Hospital: John E. Hall, MD, James R. Kasser, MD, John B. Emans, and Peter M. Waters. I strive to provide the type of care they practice and teach.

I would like to acknowledge my associates at North Shore Orthopaedic Surgery and Sports Medicine, PC, including Sanford C. Scheman, MD, Charles J. Bleifeld, MD, Gerald S. Wertleib,

MD, Kevin G. Vesey, MD, Richard A. Weiss, MD, Sandra J. Ianotti, MD, and Mark J. Sterling, MD for being great doctors and for always supporting me in my endeavors. Similar regards are extended to other colleagues including David M. Hirsh, MD, Roy G. Kulick, MD, Monroe N. Szporn, MD and Julian G. Sallis, MD.

I am thankful to both Laurence and Jacqueline Weitzman who not only believed me when I said I was going to write this book but were crucial in helping me along the way. I would also like to acknowledge the valuable assistance of Michael Goldberg.

I am grateful to my distinguished colleagues who reviewed the book or individual chapters: Charles J. Bleifeld, MD, Nathan H. Lebwohl, MD, and Edward S. Crane, MD.

Neeti Madan is an extraordinary agent. I want to thank her and Tracy Bernstein, my editor, and New American Library, my publisher, for believing in this book and working so hard to make it happen.

Thanks to all of my dear friends and wonderful family. I am lucky to have each and every one of you.

Finally, but most importantly, I would like to thank my wife, Mindy, for her patience, support, love, amazing last-minute editing skills, and for giving birth to the greatest gift of all, our son, Ethan Sy.

CONTENTS

Section II:
THE CAUSES OF BACK PAIN

Section IV:
GOING UNDER THE KNIFE:
Surgical Procedures

Section V:
AFTER THE SURGERY:
Care and Complications

INTRODUCTION

Everyone experiences back pain. If you haven't yet, just wait a few years. If you have, you know that it can be a life-altering problem. At its worst, it can make even the simplest daily activities—walking, lifting, bending—painful or even impossible. When that happens, the idea of having surgery to make the pain go away is very alluring. You just go to the doctor, and he runs some tests. He finds the problem, he operates, and you're cured. Simple, right? Unfortunately, it doesn't always work that way.

There are conditions for which surgery is not only appropriate but necessary; but there are also conditions that don't respond as well to surgery, and telling the difference between the two is what this book is all about. A case in point is chronic low back pain. The odds of curing it with surgery remain uncertain, yet every year almost half a million patients try some kind of invasive or surgical procedure to stop the pain. They all believe their problem is the kind that surgery can fix, although there's compelling evidence that it often isn't. So why are more and more people getting back surgery? The answer is complicated, and involves the surgeon, the patient, and the back itself.

THE SURGEON

If there is evidence that back surgery doesn't always work for low back pain, why do so many surgeons do it? The single most important reason is that surgeons are trained to fix people and they naturally want to use the tools they have to make people feel better. Spinal surgery works wonders for serious problems like a broken bone or disc material crushing a nerve. And so, when someone shows up on a surgeon's doorstep in agonizing pain from an arthritic disc and asks for assistance, the surgeon is inclined to do whatever he can.

The problem is that the "whatever" may not be as helpful as we once thought. The only way to tell if surgery has helped patients is to do some kind of research into how they fared. For a long time, there wasn't a lot of rigorous, reliable research coming out of the spine field (and to see what I mean by rigorous and reliable, see the note that follows on evidence). More is coming out now, but the fact is that top-quality research hasn't kept up with advances in the field.

The last two decades have seen the development of breathtaking new surgical techniques and sophisticated spinal implants. Spinal surgeons now have complete access to the spine: we can get to it from the front, the side, and the back; we can even get to the front from the back! Some researchers have correlated a recent increase in the rates of spinal fusion for low back pain to the FDA approval in 1996 of spinal fusion cages.[i] These and other devices permit a surgeon to realign and fuse the spine into a new position. But having a new technique, a new tool, or a new implant doesn't always mean pain is cured. A critical analysis of trends in spinal surgery of the past twenty years observed that: "Although a shift toward a greater use of technology was noted . . . the clinical benefit of this trend remains unclear."[ii] We have come to a point where there is a mismatch between our surgical skills and techniques and our knowledge of how best to use them to cure back pain.

Surgeons are beginning to understand this and some are becoming more cautious about recommending certain surgical procedures. Six prominent surgeons published a 2003 article about treating low back pain in the medical journal *Spine*. It examined the efficacy of the most common surgical procedures used to treat low back pain, and concluded that:

> It should be emphasized that all of the aforementioned procedures for low back pain have unpredictable outcomes; therefore, these procedures should be only considered after failure of conservative therapy of at least 6 months and with the full understanding of patients who are well informed about the potential advantages, disadvantages, and unpredictable outcomes. *It is not established in the literature that any of these procedures, including fusion techniques, are superior to natural history or nonoperative treatment.*[iii] (italics mine)

Note the key phrase "natural history," which is what doctors say when they mean "doing nothing." The gist of the article is that surgery for chronic low back pain hasn't been shown to be better than other options.

And so treating back pain has proved to be much more complicated than most patients and doctors expected. Thinking that you can show up at your surgeon's office and he will recommend a surgical procedure that will instantly cure your pain is an unrealistic expectation. This is why patients need to take an active role in both the diagnosis and treatment of their back problems.

THE PATIENT

When a patient walks into a doctor's office, the deck is stacked against him. He's meeting with a guy in a white coat with a whole bunch of diplomas on the wall. The chronic pain he's been enduring for months or years makes him more susceptible than usual to the promise, or even the possibility, of relief. He's eager to find something—anything—to make his back stop hurting, and naturally he wants his doctor to help him.

In my experience, patients are often unwilling to second-guess doctors who recommend surgery, and sometimes even protest when doctors *don't* recommend surgery. I've seen patients who, in the face of all the evidence and the recommendations of several doctors, are convinced that surgery—and only surgery—will fix their problems. Maybe it's because their aunt Sally had a similar problem that surgery fixed; maybe they read about it on the Internet; maybe they saw an ad for a particular procedure. They're true believers.

I understand how it happens. Patients are looking for a way to stop the pain, and surgery is awfully tempting. It doesn't require them to undertake a long, and sometimes uncomfortable, regimen of physical therapy. It doesn't require them to get regular exercise. And it doesn't require them to find another doctor who has a solution other than surgery. Even though surgery may not be the best long-term answer, it's simple. When you're in pain, what you want more than anything else is for someone to make it go away, and that desire grows stronger with every round of unsuccessful nonsurgical treatment. I've seen many patients who feel as though they've tried everything else, and they come to me almost in desperation, with the strong conviction that surgery is the only answer. Often, though, they've been trying the wrong things, or the right things in the wrong combination, or potential right things that just need a little more time to work.

CASE STUDY

Since college, TONY, a forty-eight-year-old furniture maker, had occasional, but manageable, backaches. A year or so before he came to me, they started to get progressively worse, and he went to see a spinal surgeon. After an MRI scan showed a degenerated disc, he was given a prescription for codeine and physical therapy. He thought therapy sounded like a great idea, since he'd put on some weight and was too busy and stressed to find the time to exercise on his own. His therapy, though, consisted more of hot packs and ultrasound than exercise, and didn't help his pain. He went back to the surgeon, who found that a second MRI scan showed a herniated disc in addition to the degenerated disc, and recommended a laminectomy and spinal fusion. Tony was relieved to hear that there was a cure for the pain that was taking such a toll on his job and his life. When he came to me for a second opinion, he told me that all nonsurgical treatments had failed, and that surgery was the only option. It took some doing to convince him that there were options he hadn't tried that were as likely as surgery—and perhaps more likely than surgery—to alleviate his pain. Four months into a program of exercise and physical therapy, and fifteen pounds lighter, Tony had his back pain well under control.

While not every case of back pain responds the way Tony's did, Tony's experience, with its wrong turns and delays, is very common. This book will help you zero in on the kinds of treatment that are most likely to work, and skip the kinds that won't. If you find effective nonsurgical treatment early, you're much less likely to get to the desperation phase of back pain, when surgery seems like the only option. To make the right treatment choices, you have to start by understanding the complicated, maddening, poorly understood structure that is the source of all the problems that led me to write this book: the back itself.

THE BACK

There's a lot about back pain we simply don't understand. Most instances of surgery that don't work out follow a similar pattern. A patient has pain, and the surgeon runs tests that reveal some kind of abnormality in the spine. The surgeon performs a procedure to correct the abnormality, the patient recovers, but the pain doesn't go away. Sometimes the surgery results in even more pain.

The biggest reason this happens is very straightforward. That abnormality—the one you just had surgically corrected—may not have been causing the pain that drove you to the surgeon.

About thirty-five percent of all forty-year-olds have at least one degenerated disc that shows up on an MRI, and many of them have no back pain at all.[iv] The idea that a degenerated disc may not be the source of pain seems difficult for both patient and doctor to accept. Way back in 1990, Dr. Scott Haldeman, then president of the North American Spine Society, saw the problem coming. In his presidential address, he voiced a prescient concern that the very human desire for certainty would lead to an increasing trend in inappropriate surgery. "Physicians and patients tend to feel more comfortable with a clear-cut relationship between pathology and symptomatology, between health and disease, and between cause and effect."[v]

Abnormalities on tests are often unrelated to back pain. Many people over a certain age—about forty—get back pain. Lots of people that age also have some kind of spine abnormality. The problem is that the abnormality is rarely the source of the pain.

Take, for instance, the case of herniated discs. While there are some kinds of pain (sciatica, primarily) that can be reliably pegged to a herniated disc and alleviated with surgery, there are other kinds that most definitely can't. Of course, when an adult over forty *with* back pain has a herniated disc, it's tempting to conclude that the disc is causing the pain. But then how do we explain all those adults who are walking around with herniated discs and *no* back pain? The 2003 *Spine* article addresses the difficulty of answering that question:

> The clinicians' challenge in treating patients with persistent low back pain is the absence of a test to accurately diagnose discogenic pain and the absence of reliable patient selection criteria favoring a good outcome. . . . More research to determine the pathogenesis of disc degeneration and the mechanism or source of low back pain will guide the logical choice of therapeutic strategies or interventions in the future.[vi]

In other words, finding the source of pain can be difficult, and it is dangerous to seize on a lump on an MRI as the culprit. We often can't tell where pain is coming from, and we need to do more research to find ways to do it better. In the meantime, one of the things my patients find most difficult to accept is that the answer to their most basic question, "What's causing my pain?"

is all too often, "We don't know for sure." They have to go to a *doctor* to hear that? The patient's first impulse is to find another doctor, a better doctor, to tell him what's wrong. I'm sorry to say that I have had many patients who, frustrated with my recommendation against surgery, found another doctor who was willing to operate. Sometimes they came back with pain worsened by the surgery they sought. That doesn't mean that there is no help for your back pain. It does mean that in order to find the best solution for you, you need to fully understand what choices are available.

WHY THIS BOOK?

Back pain is a complex problem with an equally complex set of treatment options. This book is designed to help you make the match between your particular problem and the treatment options most likely to work for you. Sometimes, that's a straightforward process. Where diagnoses are definitive and treatment is well established, I'll just give you the basics. Where doctors disagree, and treatments are unpredictable, I'll go into much more detail and help you decide which side you should be on.

In short, I want to show you what you're up against and prepare you to deal with it. I've been operating on backs for over fifteen years and I've seen both remarkable successes and unnecessary failures. The bottom line is that a patient who is well informed has the best chance of finding the most effective treatment. The goal of this book is to help you be that patient.

ENDNOTES

i R. A. Deyo, D. T. Gray, W. Kreuter, et al., "United States Trends in Lumbar Fusion Surgery for Degenerative Conditions," *Spine* 30, no. 12 (2005), pp. 1441–45.

ii C. M. Bono, C. K. Lee, "Critical Analysis of Trends in Fusion for Degenerative Disc Disease Over the Past 20 Years: Influence of Technique on Fusion Rate and Clinical Outcome," *Spine* 29, no. 4 (2004), pp. 455–63.

iii H. An, S. D. Boden, J. Kang, et al., "Summary Statement: Emerging Techniques for Treatment of Degenerative Lumbar Disc Disease," *Spine* 28, no. 15S (2003), pp. S24–25.

iv S. D. Boden, et al., "Abnormal Magnetic-Resonance Scans of the Lumbar Spine in Asymptomatic Subjects: A Prospective Investigation," *Journal of Bone and Joint Surgery* (Am.) 72-A, no. 3 (1990): pp. 403–8.

v S. Haldeman, "North American Spine Society: Failure of the Pathology Model to Predict Back Pain," *Spine* 15, no. 7 (1990), pp. 718–24.

vi H. An, et al., "Summary Statement."

AUTHOR'S NOTE ON SCIENTIFIC EVIDENCE AND BACK PAIN

The recommendations I make in this book are based on what I think all doctors' recommendations should be based on: evidence. In medicine, that comes from research. All research is not created equal, though; a large part of sorting through evidence is assessing its quality.

The highest-quality evidence comes from what scientists call prospective, placebo-controlled, randomized, double-blind studies, so I want to explain what those are. "Prospective" means that the study begins before patients have gotten the treatment. (The opposite is retrospective, which looks at a group of people who have already had the treatment to see how they fared.) "Placebo-controlled" means that the group that gets the real treatment is compared to a group that gets a sham treatment that seems as similar as possible to the real treatment. "Randomized" means that patients are assigned to the treatment group or the control group at random. "Double-blind" means that neither the patients nor the researchers know who's in which group.

When possible, I rely on research like that in my discussions on the efficacy of surgical and nonsurgical treatments. Sometimes, though, it doesn't exist. High-quality clinical trials are expensive, difficult to coordinate, and time-consuming. There are also problems with double-blinding and placebo-controlling, particularly if it's a surgical technique that's being studied. It's not possible to design a study so that the patient doesn't know whether he's had spinal fusion.

Although research that's retrospective, unblinded, uncontrolled, or all three isn't as valuable, it's not useless. If, after the fact, we look back at a large group of patients who've had a particular treatment for a particular condition and find that most of them have fared poorly, that's a pretty good indication that we should be looking for better ways to handle that condition. It doesn't tell us whether they would have done better with another treatment, or no treatment at all, but it does tell us that the treatment they got isn't great.

There's so much research, and so many statistics, that it's difficult to know how much to tell you. Some readers, no doubt, will want to know the details. What percent got better? After how long? With what complication rate? Others will want an executive summary.

As I said, I will vary the level of detail according to how controversial the issue is. If everyone, or almost everyone, in the field agrees, I stick to a brief summary of the data. You won't find too many numbers in the section on exercise (good for the back) or bed rest (bad for the back). The section on fusion surgery for back pain, though, has a lot of detail. I know that, for some of you, it will be too much, and, for others, too little. If you're one of the former, rest assured that I also give an executive summary. If you're one of the latter, you'll find refuge in the endnotes, which will tell you where you can go for more information.

The point of parsing the research isn't to tell you that a particular procedure has a 67.5 percent chance of solving your particular problem. The point is to tell you whether the chance of success is good or not good, and whether it's better or worse than another treatment. That's the best that evidence can do, but that can take you a long way toward making the right decision.

THE
BACK
STORY

The Basics of Spines and Surgery

Chapter 1

A SPINE TUTORIAL

S pines are complicated. They support us, they give us mobility, and they house our spinal nerves. Sometimes these three functions are at odds. In order to keep us upright, a spine needs to be stable, but to let us do everything from tying our shoes to lifting our luggage into the overhead compartment, it needs to be flexible. While doing all that, it also has to protect the spinal cord, which runs through it and provides the conduit for sensations to reach the brain and for the brain's messages to reach our limbs. That's a lot to ask from one structure.

To complicate issues, conversations about the spine are peppered with unfamiliar, difficult-to-pronounce words (spondylolisthesis, anyone?). So before we go into what can go wrong with spines, and what to do about it, I want to cover the basics. Once you have a good working knowledge of spine anatomy, it's much easier to understand things like spondylolisthesis, and everything else in this book. It's also much easier to talk to your doctor and to read other medical literature. You can't make good decisions without a solid understanding, and that understanding starts here.

This is inevitably a simplification of a very complex part of your body. I've tried to include everything you need to know to make informed decisions about back treatments without cluttering it up with what you probably don't need to know. Think of it as Spine 101.

THE SPINE IN FULL

Here it is, from top to bottom.

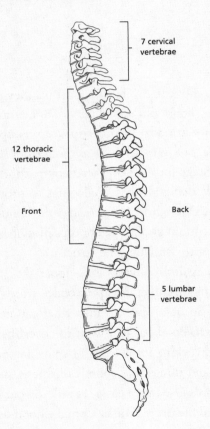

7 cervical
vertebrae

12 thoracic
vertebrae

Front

Back

5 lumbar
vertebrae

Side view of the entire spine showing the bones (vertebrae) and the normal curvatures including lumbar lordosis, thoracic kyphosis and cervical lordosis.

The top part is the cervical spine, which consists of the first seven vertebrae, beginning at the back of your neck. The middle part is the thoracic spine, the twelve vertebrae directly below. Below the thoracic spine are the five vertebrae of the lumbar spine. Below that are the sacrum and coccyx, which form part of the pelvis.

Things can go wrong anywhere along the spine, but most back problems happen in the lumbar spine, which is why this book deals almost exclusively with those five troublesome vertebrae.

THE SUM OF ITS PARTS
The Vertebra

Reach behind you and run your fingers down your spine. Feel those bumps? Each bump is part of a vertebra, and your spine consists of a long line of them.

The vertebrae are all labeled according to their position in your spine. The five vertebrae that make up the lumbar spine are labeled, unimaginatively but clearly, L1 to L5, where L1 is closest to your neck and L5 is closest to your tailbone. The cervical and thoracic spines are labeled the same way: C1 to C7 and T1 to T12 respectively.

The vertebrae that make up the cervical and thoracic portions of the spine look a little different from lumbar vertebrae, and different from each other. Because this book is about low back problems, I'm only going to show you what a lumbar vertebra looks like.

Although a vertebra is one piece of bone, it's a complex piece, and many of its parts have their own names. When we talk about those parts, we tend to refer to them as though they were distinct bones, as in, "Spondylolysis is a fracture of the

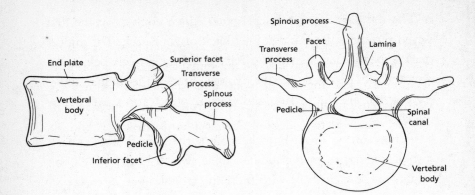

A lumbar vertebrae: side view (left) and top down (right).

pars interarticularis." Or, "A laminectomy removes all or part of the lamina." Those terms are very convenient because they let us refer very specifically to a small part of the vertebra, but those parts aren't quite as well defined as their Latin names make them sound. I can't show you precisely where the lamina ends and the spinous process begins, but I can come close enough.

Here are the parts of the vertebra.

Vertebral Body

This is the big cylindrical section that abuts the discs above and below. It looks like a uniform piece of bone, but it's not. It's a little like an egg, with a hard shell on the outside made of what you think of when you think of bone—the hard stuff called cortical bone. Inside that shell is much softer material called cancellous bone, or bone marrow. The top and the bottom of the cylinder also have a layer called the end plate, which is a combination of cartilage and bone. Attached to the back of the vertebral body is a ring of bone with many parts, each of which has its own name.

Pedicle

These are the parts of the ring directly connected to the vertebral body, and they form the sides of the spinal canal. There are two, one on each side. You need to know about pedicles if you're considering a fusion with pedicle screw instrumentation, because this is where many doctors choose to connect hardware to the bone.

Transverse Process

If you travel around the bony ring starting at the vertebral body, this is the first pointy structure you will encounter. There's one on either side, sticking out from your spine pointing to the side. One type of spinal fusion is done from the back (posterolateral) and involves laying a bone graft over these structures to immobilize (or fuse) part of the spine.

Facets

The facets are the four protrusions that connect each vertebra to its neighbors. In doing so, they keep the spine aligned. Two facets join with the vertebra above (those are called the superior facets), and two with the vertebra below (the inferior facets). The point where two facets meet is called the facet joint. The facets are covered with cartilage the same way the bones of your knees and hips are. The cartilage reduces friction so the joints move smoothly and the bones don't wear down. But wait, there's more! The joint is also surrounded by a capsule containing a lubricant called synovial fluid, your spine's answer to WD-40. Between the cartilage and the synovial fluid, the movement of your facet is almost frictionless.

Facet joints, like other joints, are vulnerable to arthritis, and an arthritic facet joint can be painful, and, in more extreme circumstances, can allow one of your vertebrae to slip in front of the other because it's no longer able to keep the vertebrae properly aligned.

Pars Interarticularis

This is the part that connects the superior and inferior facets above and below the vertebra. The pars (we often drop the "interarticularis" when we talk about it) is susceptible to stress fractures, which, depending on their severity, can cause pain or instability.

Lamina

There are two for each vertebra, and they form the back of the spinal canal, where they join in the middle and connect to the spinous process. They also provide the easiest surgical access to the spinal canal. If I need to get into it, I can remove part of the lamina (laminectomy) and work through it.

Spinous Process

This is the part of the vertebra you know best, because it's the only part you can feel. The bumps that run down your back are the ends of the spinous process. There is only one for each vertebra.

Although these parts form a shape that is roughly a ring, we refer to the vertebra as having a front and a back. The front is the vertebral body, and the back is everything else except the pedicle, which connects the front to the back.

THE PARTS THAT ARE HOLES

Just as important as bones are the places where the bones aren't. The holes in the vertebrae, and between vertebrae, are where the nerves run.

The Spinal Canal

Each vertebra has a big hole right in the middle, and when the vertebrae are stacked, one on top of the other, the holes line up and create an empty tube like an elevator shaft down your spine. The spinal cord and nerves run down that elevator shaft, and the space that's left is called the epidural space.

Neural Foramen

This is the hole between the two pedicles from adjacent vertebrae. They are formed when the vertebrae are stacked and are where the spinal nerves leave the canal. You're probably getting the idea that "foramen" is a fancy word for hole. It is.

THE DISC

Its long name is the intervertebral disc. It is the structure that separates each of the vertebral bodies. The disc is analogous to the white cream between the two chocolate wafers in an Oreo cookie, where the wafers are the vertebrae. It's a critical part of the spine, and the part that is often suspected of causing problems that don't seem to have their origins elsewhere.

The disc looks solid, but it isn't. It's constructed a lot like a jelly donut. It has a firm outer shell (called the annulus fibrosis) and a soft inner core (called the nucleus pulposus). The job of the nucleus (the jelly) is to absorb shock. Just as the hydraulic fluid in your car's shock absorbers prevent you from feeling every bump in the road, the soft inner core of your disc provides the give that prevents your vertebrae from rattling against each other with every step you take. The job of the annulus (the

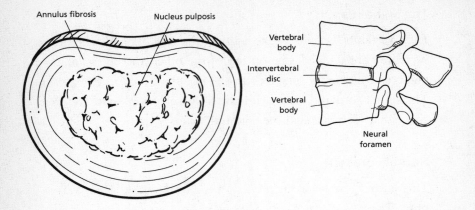

The intervertebral disc: on the left is a top-down view showing the nucleus pulposis (inside) and the annulus fibrosis (outside); and on the right is a side view in its normal position between two vertebrae.

bready part of the donut) is to keep the nucleus from leaking out, and to attach to the end plates of the vertebral bodies above and below. The annulus may play a role in back pain because there are nerves in it (there are none in the nucleus), and an annular tear might damage those nerves. We don't know for sure, though.

Like the vertebrae, the discs have simple labels. The disc between your second and third lumbar vertebrae is called the L2-L3 disc.

THE SPINAL CORD

This is the bundle of nerves that connects the brain to the rest of the body. The nerves start (or end, depending on how you look

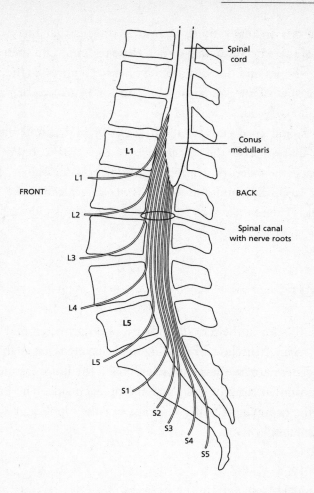

Spinal
cord

Conus
medullaris

FRONT

BACK

L1

L1

L2

L3

L4

L5

L5

S1

S2

S3

S4

S5

Spinal canal
with nerve roots

Side view of the lumbar spine with the lower end of the spinal cord,
the conus medullaris, the cauda equina and the spinal nerves.

at it) in your brain, run down your back in the spinal canal, and
branch out at every level, exiting the spine through the neural
foramina, the spaces between vertebrae. One of the reasons the
spine is important is that it has to protect these nerves. One of

the reasons so many things can go wrong is that there are so many of these nerves living in such close proximity to such structures as bones and discs. If a bone or disc compresses the spinal cord or one of the spinal nerves, pain or neurological damage can occur or both.

The spinal cord ends at about the level of L1, and then the nerves split off from the center and exit the spinal canal through the spaces between the vertebrae (the neural foramina). Below the L1 level, the bundle of nerves is no longer called the spinal cord; it is called the cauda equina (because it looks like a horse's tail).

MUSCLES

There are a lot of them in the vicinity, and they often play a role in back pain. Muscles surrounding the spine are what enable it to move. There are two large muscles, called the iliopsoas muscles, that run down the front of the spine on each side. The back of the spine has many smaller muscles, but they look and act like one big muscle.

LIGAMENTS

There are two important ligaments running the length of your spine. There's one on the front of the vertebral body, called the anterior longitudinal ligament (ALL), and one on the back of the vertebral body, inside the spinal canal, called the posterior longitudinal ligament (PLL). There are also smaller ligaments at every level of your spine. There are ones that hold the laminae together (ligamentum flavum), and there are others that attach the spinous processes to one another.

Taken together, the muscles and ligaments are an integral part of the system, and it's not surprising that they're at the root of some spine problems.

There's much more to the spine than what's in this chapter, but this will give you enough of an anatomical grounding to understand what's in the rest of the book. Don't worry about remembering it all right now; if you get to the fusion chapter and you can't quite remember where the transverse process is, you can always flip back to this section. It's not going anywhere, so forge ahead.

Chapter 2

THE PROBLEM OF PAIN: *WHAT WE DON'T KNOW*

Most of the time, the one and only way a back problem makes itself known is with pain. There's no itching, no nausea, no fever. No swelling, no redness, no palpitations. There's very little I can measure (like a pulse) or observe (like a rash). The first, and sometimes the only, clue I have to lead me to a diagnosis is my patient's description of his pain.

That leaves me, and every other back doctor, at a disadvantage, in part because the experience of pain is subjective. Have you ever sat in a room and been perfectly comfortable while the person sitting next to you thinks it's too hot, or too cold, or too humid, or that there's a funny smell? Pain works the same way; one patient's unbearable is another patient's inconvenient, and one patient's twinge is another patient's spasm. There's no such thing as an accurate assessment of pain, and that leaves me with little to go on.

That's not even the biggest problem. Even if I get a pretty good picture of the intensity and type of pain, that picture doesn't tell me nearly enough to arrive at a diagnosis. Most kinds of pain could lead me to any one of many different diagnoses, and finding the true cause of pain is almost always difficult and often impossible. Yes, there's that bad word: "impossible." Given what we know about spines, a diagnosis for the source of low back pain is often a guess. In 2001, the *New England Journal of Medicine* published an overview of low back pain that concluded that "perhaps 85% of patients with isolated low back pain cannot be given a precise pathoanatomical diagnosis."[i] Don't let the word "pathoanatomical" throw you—it just means the part of your anatomy that's responsible for the pain. If the authors weren't writing for a medical journal, they might have rephrased their conclusion along these lines: we don't know what causes most low back pain.

Although tests like MRIs and X-rays (which are all explained in detail in chapter 6) can be invaluable in diagnosis, they can also be part of the problem. They reveal physical abnormalities that can lead me down a blind alley. Many people over forty have both some back pain *and* an abnormality that shows up on a test, but the abnormality doesn't necessarily cause the pain. I mentioned this issue in the introduction, and I want to talk more about it here because it's one of the main reasons back treatment goes wrong. When I see a patient with pain, and a darkened or bulging disc shows up on an MRI, it's very, very easy to conclude that the two are connected. Often, though, people with those same abnormalities have no pain at all. Estimates vary widely, but somewhere between one-quarter and three-quarters of people with pain-free backs have a bulging or herniated disc that gets picked up on an MRI.

A lot of this book details what we know about backs and how they respond to surgery, but this chapter—and it's a critical one—is about what we *don't* know and how to deal with uncertainty. I admit that if you're a patient with low back pain, you'll read a lot of what's in this chapter as bad news. But there's good news, too. I'm going to give you a new way to think about low back pain that should help you treat the pain effectively and significantly reduce the odds that you'll be tempted by inappropriate surgery.

> **Everything connects: the spine, the mind, and the pain.** One study recruited forty-six people with no back pain and followed them for four years. At the beginning of the study, the subjects underwent testing that showed abnormalities in some of them. At the end of four years, the researchers found that those abnormalities were only a weak predictor of who got back pain. There were, however, two factors that did predict who got back pain: certain psychological indicators and chronic pain somewhere other than the lower back.[ii]

THE APPENDICITIS MODEL

Accepting uncertainty is something many of my patients have a hard time with, in part because we're all used to going to doctors who can tell us what's wrong and fix the problem. It's the appendicitis model of medicine: there's a surefire solution to an easily identifiable problem. When a patient shows up in a doctor's office with severe abdominal pain, we can run a few simple tests to tell us whether it's appendicitis or not. If it is, we remove the appendix. The pain is gone, the complications are few, the problem is fixed. It's the symptom-diagnosis-treatment model we're all comfortable with.

This approach is very appealing, and it's the kind of process most of my patients expect to go through when they make an appointment to see me. It's natural for a patient to expect a doctor to cure him, and the appendicitis model lets him put his problem squarely on someone else's shoulders. The idea that it's your doctor's job to find what's wrong with you and fix it puts you in a passive role, and I find that many of my patients expect their role in the treatment of back pain to be just that. They want to sit back and watch me do the healing. And I don't blame them. When I hire a lawyer or an accountant or a subcontractor I expect him to do the job while I do a little advising here, a little questioning there. I'm hiring someone else to do something I can't do (or don't want to do) myself.

In reality, though, the uncertainties of back pain make the appendicitis model inapplicable most of the time, and I'm going to propose an entirely new model for thinking about low back pain. Instead of thinking of the process as symptom-diagnosis-treatment, and your doctor's job, think of it simply as symptom-treatment, and as an active partnership between you and your doctor. I want you to take the diagnosis out of the loop, because that's where so much treatment goes wrong.

I want to be very clear that the problems that bring patients to spine surgeons aren't always undiagnosable. There are circumstances where a diagnosis isn't only possible but essential. Those circumstances are truly dangerous conditions for which treatment is necessary, and I cover them in chapter 5: Spine-One-One. If you've got back pain, the very first thing you need to do is rule these out.

Beyond those urgent conditions, there are other circumstances for which a diagnosis is fairly clear and treatment is dependent on that diagnosis (the appendicitis model). If I see a patient with severe sciatica and a herniated disc, a detailed history, a thorough physical exam, and an MRI will usually tell me what I need to know to figure out whether the disc is the source of the pain. These are straightforward conditions, and there are many that have to be ruled out before you turn to the symptom-treatment model.

Most of the time, though, for patients with chronic low back pain, none of these conditions is the culprit, and the symptom-treatment model is the best friend you have, because it will make you stop focusing on what's causing your pain and start focusing on how to stop it. There are two very good reasons to do this. First, we probably can't say what's causing your pain anyway. Second, even if we could, it wouldn't change the way we treat the pain.

The bottom line is that I'm asking you to forget about what's "wrong" with you. Chances are, you'd never find out definitively even if you made the search your life's work. So why bother? The objective is to make the pain go away.

Let me walk you through the process. Let's say a patient—I'll call him Steve—comes to see me for a second opinion on what to do about his chronic low back pain. He's also got a little referred pain into the buttock, but no shooting pain down his legs. His MRI results show two black discs (you'll learn all about those in chapter 6). The discs may or may not be the source of his pain; even if they are, surgery might or might not help him. The good news is that there are many treatments short of surgery that can help, whether or not the disc is the source of the pain, so once I rule out emergencies like cancer, broken bones, and infections, I don't waste my time, Steve's time, or any more resources trying to figure out exactly where the pain is coming from. I'm treating the pain, not the disc or the facet joint or the bone spur. I'm trying to get the pain to go away, and pinpointing the pain's source wouldn't tell me which of many approaches will work best. My best—arguably my only—option is to treat the symptom.

When Steve sat down in my office, he was hoping I could tell him exactly what was wrong with him and what we could do about it. I explain that it's unlikely we'll find an absolutely certain diagnosis, but that's okay because *the treatment is the same regardless*.

That treatment generally begins with modification of activity, anti-inflammatories, and physical therapy, which is where I'd start. I won't even think about trying anything more serious until he gives that six to eight weeks, or even a little more time. During that time, I'll encourage Steve to try a number of alternative therapies. Yoga helps many back patients, as does acupuncture. Many of my patients swear by chiropractics. Some are helped by the combination of glucosamine and chondroitin. Walking can help alleviate back pain (although, in some circumstances, it can also aggravate it). Some patients try swimming or cycling. I don't know which, if any, of these will work for Steve, but I do know that the more of them he tries, the better his chances of improving. It's trial and error, but it's almost risk-free.

After three months, if Steve's pain is worse, I'll start experimenting with other medication. I'll try different anti-inflammatories and various analgesics (another word for pain medication). Anti-seizure and antidepression medications have both been used successfully for chronic pain. Something as simple as a sleeping pill can help; a good night's sleep can make a difference. Some of my patients are reluctant to try a lot of different medications, and I understand their hesitation. I don't prescribe them lightly. (I take particular care with narcotics—more on that in chapter 10.) Compared to surgery, though, medication is a walk in the park.

The point is that there are many, many ways to treat back pain, and we don't have to know exactly what's wrong to try them. If none of those options work, Steve and I may try digging deeper to find out if there is a possibility of a diagnosis treatable by surgery, but most of the Steves who walk into my office never get to this point. The chances are very good that one of the alternatives, or maybe several in combination, work well enough to keep even patients with severe pain from considering surgery.

PAIN AND YOUR BRAIN

When pain is the most important, or the only, clue to what's wrong with a spine, the diagnostic process is complicated by the interaction between body and brain. I've already mentioned the problem of subjectivity, but it goes much deeper than that. We're just beginning to scratch the surface of what causes pain and what influences how we perceive it in the brain.

One thing that affects the experience of pain is expectation. If one person is told something won't hurt much and the other is told that it will hurt a lot, those expectations are borne out in their experience of pain. The person who's told it won't be so bad finds that—surprise!—it isn't so bad. Meanwhile, the unfortunate subject who's told it'll be very bad finds that it is just that. One study of patients with low back pain had them perform a simple test that involved repetitively bending the knee against resistance until they couldn't do it anymore. Some were told it would be a pain-free experience, and others were told it might hurt a little.

The subjects who expected pain not only felt it but performed the test significantly less well than the control group. They did fewer repetitions with less force and a smaller range of motion.[iii]

Expectations also come into play with pain relief. The placebo effect is particularly pronounced for chronic pain of all kinds, and back pain is no exception. This complicates not only the treatment of individual patients but also the research on how effective different back treatments are. If the patient believes the treatment will work, the chances are good that it will, at least to some degree, and at least in the short term.

One interesting aspect of the placebo effect is that not all placebos are created equal. Pills taken several times a day elicit a bigger response than pills taken only once. Shots elicit a stronger response than pills. The more powerful subjects expect the treatment to be (and if it hurts, or it's uncomfortable, or it tastes bad, it seems more powerful), the more pronounced the placebo effect is. The expectations for surgery are very high. It's reasonable to suppose that the placebo effect is commensurately high. It's very difficult, though, to assess the strength of surgery's placebo effect. Researching it requires putting subjects through fake-operations, complete with anesthesia and incisions; it's an enterprise fraught with ethical peril.

We can put science around a lot of the reasons people get better if they expect to get better, but many years of treating different kinds of people has taught me that intangibles also matter. I have seen patients who come to me with identical problems and have identical treatments but end up with very different results. I can only hazard a guess that recovery from an injury or disease is also based on attitude, outlook, and other aspects of personality and worldview that I can't even put my finger on.

Every patient has to understand that treating pain is a tricky business even under the best of circumstances. Although pain is now being considered a vital sign, like pulse and body temperature, it can't be measured with a watch or a thermometer. The only person who can gauge pain is the person experiencing it, so doctors have to work from what is essentially secondhand information. Pain also varies with attitude, expectation, and personality. When the pain is in the back, the process is further complicated by the complexity of the spine and the huge variety of problems that *might* be the pain's source. All of this adds up to uncertainty, which is what every back patient has to expect as he embarks with his doctor on the trial-and-error process of alleviating pain.

Eventually, for some patients, that trial-and-error process culminates in surgery. For most conditions, though, surgery is either a last resort or not an option. Because we simply don't know enough about backs to make definitive diagnoses every time, the first solutions to try are the least risky or invasive. If a patient embarks on, say, a regimen of exercise and Tylenol, the worst-case scenario is that it doesn't help the pain. If a patient has a complicated spinal reconstructive surgery, the worst case is as bad as worst cases can be.

As you start the process of treating your back pain, I want to help you set your expectations realistically and constructively. That will enable you to navigate the world of doctors and treatments effectively and, hopefully, successfully. So expect uncertainty. Expect frustration. Expect trial and error. But also expect to get better. Expect that you will find a treatment—probably a nonsurgical one—that will get your pain under control and free you to get back to your life.

ENDNOTES

i R. A. Deyo, J. N. Weinstein, "Low Back Pain," *New England Journal of Medicine* 344, no. 5 (2001), pp. 363–70.

ii E. J. Carragee, et al., "Prospective Controlled Study of the Development of Lower Back Pain in Previously Asymptomatic Subjects Undergoing Experimental Discography," *Spine* 29, no. 10 (2004), pp. 1112–17.

iii M. Pfingsten, et al., "Fear-Avoidance Behavior and Anticipation of Pain in Patients With Chronic Low Back Pain: A Randomized Controlled Study," *Pain Medicine* 2, no. 4 (2001), pp. 259–66.

Chapter 3

FINDING A DOCTOR

I f you think you need surgery, the smartest thing to do may be to
not look for a surgeon—at least not right away. There are lots
of circumstances when an altogether different kind of doctor
might be the best place to begin. There are doctors who specialize
in pain management, nerve disorders, and physical therapy who
can help a patient with back pain try nonsurgical approaches. If
your mind-set is that you're treating *pain*, rather than a degenerated disc or an internal disc disruption or any other specific diagnosis, it makes sense to try them first. Unless you're really
determined to have surgery, it doesn't make any sense to rush to a
surgeon.

Start with your primary care physician, and work with her to
first figure out what kind of doctor you should see and, then,
which specific doctor.

Let's start with what kind of doctor. There are several nonsurgical choices.

Physiatrist: You may not be aware that there is such a thing as
a physiatrist, but I advise many of my patients to get to know
one. Physiatrists specialize in physical medicine (the mechanics
of your body) and rehabilitation, which is why they're also
known as PM&R. Their reason for being is to help you avoid

surgery, and their tools range from physical therapy to pain management strategies.

Neurologist: Not to be confused with a neurosurgeon (who does the actual surgery), a neurologist deals with disorders and diseases of the nerves. You should consider a consultation with a neurologist if there is evidence that nerves are involved in your back problem. That evidence is sciatica (or other shooting pain), numbness, tingling, or weakness in the legs. A neurologist is a sensible first step when you want to consider nonsurgical treatment options. Even if you don't think your pain indicates nerve involvement, it may be worthwhile to consult a neurologist.

Before we move on, there is one common misconception I'd like to clear up. Many of my patients have the idea that a neurologist is something akin to a psychiatrist. That is not true. Neurologists don't treat neuroses. Although many nerve disorders involve the brain, the neurologist is not the guy who's going to put you on the proverbial couch.

Rheumatologist: Doctors who study diseases of the joints and soft tissues treat inflammatory disorders, arthritis, lupus, osteoporosis, fibromyalgia, and other related conditions. Many of them treat back pain, which often comes with the rheumatological territory. They know how to manage chronic conditions, and back pain falls into that category.

Pain management specialist: This isn't a formal category, but it encompasses all kinds of doctors who specialize in managing pain. Some neurologists and physiatrists specialize in pain management, but so do other kinds of doctors, from anesthesiologists to invasive radiologists. No matter what your back problem is, and no matter how you decide to treat it, managing pain will be an inevitable part of the process. The goal, of course, is to make it go away, so although a pain specialist should probably not be your first line of defense, you may want to see one.

With all that said, you shouldn't rule out a surgeon. There are two kinds of doctors who operate on spines: orthopedic surgeons and neurosurgeons. Orthopedic surgeons have training in bone- and joint-related problems throughout the body, and neurosurgeons specialize in the brain, spinal cord, and nerves. The specialties overlap when it comes to the spine. There's not a bright line between the two in spine surgery because many problems have roots in both specialties, and I can't give you hard-and-fast rules about which kind you should consult. Don't hesitate to see either, or both.

Both these kinds of surgeons know more about the enigma of back pain than anyone else, and either kind should be able to help you. The key is finding a surgeon who won't send you straight to the operating room without exhausting all of your other options. Which brings me to the all-important question of how to find a conservative surgeon.

First, let's talk about just what a conservative surgeon is. It's *not* someone who avoids surgery at all costs. Sometimes the conservative treatment *is* surgery. If you show up in my trauma center with a burst fracture (a bone pushing on your nerves) and weakness in your legs, I'm going to operate, and I'm about as conservative as they come. A conservative surgeon is one who, given equal evidence of efficacy, tries the less risky treatments first, and only moves on to the more risky treatments when the less risky ones prove ineffective. Alas, there is no official body rating surgeons' conservatism. You're just going to have to make an appointment and go talk about it.

Where to start looking for a surgeon? Your primary care physician is a good beginning, and I've found that word of mouth has brought a lot of my patients to me. Almost everyone has a friend or a neighbor, a cousin or a coworker, who's had experience with back doctors. Ask them about it, and you may stumble onto a great recommendation.

There are several other places you can go for referrals. Your insurance company or HMO may be helpful. Sometimes hospitals have a referral system; call around. Other doctors, even in unrelated fields, might be able to point you in the right direction; don't hesitate to ask your cardiologist, for example.

Another way to find a doctor is to follow the news in the medical field. If there's a story about a new back treatment in your local paper, read it. While the treatment may or may not be relevant to your condition, the article might very well quote doctors in your area who support or oppose it, and those quotes may give you a clue about what kind of doctors they are.

INTERNET INFORMATION

The Internet is probably where most of my patients go first, and not just to find a doctor but to find information about their condition, potential treatments, research, and support groups. It's a rich source of information, but it's a double-edged sword. While there are lots of reputable sites, there's also a lot of bunk. To find out just how much bunk, a group of orthopedic surgeons took a close look at the information on Web sites that popped up on common search engines when they entered the word "scoliosis." On only three of the fifty sites they evaluated was 75 percent or more of the information accurate. On twenty-one sites, only a quarter or less of the information was accurate.[i] That's a horrible record.

I find that the Web sites of academies or professional societies are useful and generally reliable, but there are also some good all-purpose, consumer-oriented sites. Here are some of the sites I recommend.

Professional societies for surgeons:

American Academy of Orthopaedic Surgeons
(www.aaos.org)
American Association of Neurological Surgeons
(www.aans.org)
North American Spine Society (www.spine.org)
International Society for the Study of the Lumbar Spine
(www.issls.org)
American Spinal Injury Association (www.asia-spinalinjury.org)

Other professional societies:

American Academy of Physical Medicine and Rehabilitation
(www.aapmr.org)
American Academy of Neurology (www.aan.com)
American Academy of Pain Management
(www.aapainmanage.org)
American College of Rheumatology
(www.rheumatology.org)

General-purpose sites:

Webmd.com (www.webmd.com)
MedicineNet (www.medicinenet.com)
National Institutes of Health (www.nih.gov)
The Mayo Clinic (www.mayoclinic.com)

There is one more site I want to tell you about, and it's one I rely on. It's called Pubmed, and it's a repository of virtually all the articles in all the major medical journals. Pubmed's chief asset is its comprehensiveness. If there's research on a particular topic, you'll find it on Pubmed—and there's research on just about every topic you can imagine. The downside is twofold. First, the articles are mostly written by doctors, for doctors. They're dense and jargon-ridden, and sometimes very difficult for patients to understand. Second, for most of the articles you're only given access to the abstracts, not the full text. You can often go to the Web sites of the publishers to get the full text, but it'll cost you. (If there's a medical library with public access near you, you'll be able to find most of the articles either in the stacks or online.)

One of the reasons I'm writing this book is to translate the most relevant research on backs, back pain, and surgery into ordinary English, so you don't have to try and make sense of the medicalese on Pubmed. If my experience with patients is any guide, though, I know that some of you will want to know more. If that's you, go to www.pubmed.gov. This book will not just give you a good grounding in the research that's out there, it will also give you an understanding of some of the concepts and vocabulary you'll find on Pubmed.

MEET YOUR DOCTOR

Once you've picked a doctor, there are a few simple steps that can make your initial appointment go smoothly. If you've spent a lot of time in doctors' offices lately, you know the drill. It starts with the phone call to make the appointment, and the irritating but necessary (for most of us) issue of insurance. Make sure you have your insurance information when you call, and if you need a referral from your primary care physician, make sure you have that too.

On appointment day, bring all results from any tests you've already had done—and that means both the films (X-rays) and the reports (write-ups). Also, bring whatever paperwork your insurance company requires. Bring something to read (or listen to), because chances are good you're going to have to spend some time in the waiting room or the exam room. Bring a list of the questions you'd like to ask; it's easy to forget them when you're sitting in a cold room, half naked, talking to a virtual stranger in a white coat. A lot of my patients also like to bring another human being—spouse, parent, friend—both to ask questions they might forget and to provide moral support.

The question part is important. Not only does asking the right questions get you information you need, it establishes you as your doctor's partner in the quest to ease your pain. When it comes to question asking, there are all kinds of patients. I see some who just listen and nod. On the other end of the spectrum are the ones who come with notes, lists, ideas, information, and questions, questions, questions. I'm always more comfortable with the latter, both because it makes my job easier when we're interacting like two actual people and because it gives me a hint that this patient is engaged in the process and wants to get better. And you already know that wanting to get better is a big part of getting better.

QUESTIONS, QUESTIONS

You get two kinds of information when you ask your doctor a question. The first is obvious—you get the answer to the question you ask. The second is more subtle. You get an indication of what kind of a doctor your doctor is. For starters, you'll find out if she's the kind who bridles at being asked questions. But you may also be able to find out how she views the role of you, the patient.

You can get answers to some of the basic questions about your doctor's background from the Internet, your insurance company, and the office staff. You don't have to make an appointment to find out where he went to school. These are the kinds of questions you should have no trouble finding answers to:

How many years have you been in practice?
Are you board certified or board eligible?
Did you complete a fellowship in spinal surgery?
Are you a member of any professional societies?

These are important questions about your doctor's background. You'll find out about the doctor's experience level, and something about his education. If he's board certified, he's passed a series of very rigorous tests and hurdles. If he's board eligible, he's on his way. If he's completed a fellowship in spine surgery, he's gotten very specialized training. There are many professional societies in medicine at local, state, and national levels. There are also special societies for physicians who treat spinal problems.

Once you've found a doctor, and you're further down the road to diagnosis and treatment, there are other, more specific, questions you might want to ask.

What are all of the options for treating my condition?
How much research is there about treating my condition the way you're recommending?
What has that research shown?
What are my chances for improving?

What are the risks?

What are the other options?

How do the benefits and risks of those other options compare to what you suggest?

Your doctor should have clear answers for questions like these, and others that this book will cover. Don't be afraid to ask about the research results for a particular treatment being recommended. You need to know. You shouldn't go forward with any treatment for any condition unless you get, and understand, answers to those questions.

If you're considering surgery, asking the right questions takes on particular importance. If your doctor suggests physical therapy, or pain medication, or exercise, there isn't much downside to trying it. You have everything to gain and nothing to lose; if it doesn't work, you'll try something else. Surgery, however, is an irreversible step.

Here are some of the questions you need to ask about your doctor's experience:

How long have you been performing this procedure?

How many of these procedures have you done, or do you do?

Most of my patients don't ask me questions like this, primarily because they have a sense that asking about my experience is tantamount to questioning it, or that it's just plain rude. Neither of these things is true. You probably wouldn't hesitate to ask your mechanic how long he's been fixing Toyotas, or your lawyer if he's done many incorporations, or your contractor how many kitchens he's remodeled. It should be the same with doctors. You're entitled to ask about their experience.

Other important questions are specific to your condition and the procedure you are considering:

Have I exhausted all the nonsurgical options? If not, why not?
How long will I be in the hospital?
What are the risks?
What are the risks of not having surgery?
What's the chance that I'll get better with surgery? Without it?
What do you base that assessment on?
What's the risk of needing follow-up surgery?
Will I need to go to a rehabilitation hospital after surgery?
Will I need to wear a brace? If so, for how long?

The single most important thing I can tell you about questions is that you shouldn't be afraid to ask them. Don't be afraid of offending your doctor; don't be afraid of sounding stupid; and don't be afraid of taking too much time. It's *your* back.

THE TWO-WAY INFORMATION STREET

So far, this chapter has been about getting information from your doctor, but there's also information you have to *give* her. You shouldn't worry too much about what it is; she'll ask for what she needs. But when she does, it's important that you answer her truthfully and completely. I know you may find this shocking, but patients have been known to leave out certain bits of information because they're ashamed or embarrassed. It's a natural feeling. I understand it. But that missing information could lead a surgeon in the wrong direction or compromise a surgery's success. Your doctor may ask about medications, drugs, alcohol use, incontinence and bowel function, numbness in your genital area, changes in sensitivity during sex, or difficulty in maintaining an erection. So be prepared to talk about all the things you think you are not supposed to talk about in polite company. Of course, remember that your medical record is private; it can't be shared with anyone unrelated to your medical care unless you specifically give the permission to do so.

CASE STUDY

ADAM had spinal stenosis. His problem was straightforward, and I performed a lumbar laminectomy. It all went very well; the leg pains he had been suffering virtually disappeared. He seemed, though, to suffer from a new kind of pain, originating from the incision in his back. We did the routine tests to make sure there were no complications, and I kept him in the hospital, on a morphine pain pump, for a couple of days longer than usual. Eventually, we got his pain under control and sent him home. He started calling with complaints of pain and specifically requests for more pain medication, and I started to worry that I had misdiagnosed him. I remembered an episode from my residency, when a surgeon did the same procedure on a patient, only to find out that the patient also had an unrelated neurological condition whose symptoms could mimic spinal stenosis. I sent him for an emergency MRI, which looked as it should for someone who'd just had a laminectomy. I couldn't figure out what the problem was until I called his primary care physician. It turned out that his PCP was prescribing pain medication, and had been for quite some time. In short, my patient had a Percocet habit. Before the surgery, he'd been taking more than ten pills a day, and he never told me. Had I known, I would have weaned him off it before the procedure, so his pain pill dependency wouldn't interfere with his recovery from surgery. Once I found out, we put together a plan for weaning him off the pills with the help of a pain management specialist. He's doing well; his back is fixed and he's off the Percocet.

SECOND OPINIONS

I've known people to spend more time deciding on a new computer than deciding on spine surgery. They read articles, surf the Internet, talk to computer-savvy friends, and exhaustively compare prices before they're willing to commit to a new laptop; but when a doctor suggests spine surgery, they just say "Okay."

It shouldn't be that way. Different doctors have remarkably different approaches to treating back pain, and getting a second opinion is one way to understand what your options are. Caution: I would not tell your second doctor what the first doctor suggested as treatment unless he asks. That's not to trick him, but to let him take a fresh look at your problem without being influenced by a diagnosis or treatment plan that came before. When patients come to me for second opinions, the first thing many of them tell me, even before they tell me about their problem, is what the first doctor recommended. I try to stop them before they divulge that information because I don't want to know it until I've come to my own conclusions.

When you call to make an appointment to get a second opinion, make sure you mention that that's what you're doing. A few doctors don't give second opinions as a matter of policy. It is also very important that you specifically tell your doctor, not just the office staff, that you are there for a second opinion.

If your first and second opinions are different, it might leave you confused. It seems to leave you almost worse off than you started—if doctors can't agree about what to do, how are you ever going to find a solution? You're not worse off, though. In fact, you're much better off for having established two things: first, that you have a variety of options and aren't locked into any one, and, second, that at least two options are on the table already. From there, you have a couple of choices. You can go to whichever of the doctors made the most sense to you (and suggested the less risky treatment), or you can get a third opinion to help sort things out. Either way, you're making progress. If I've done my job, you're already convinced that treating back pain is often a process of trial and error, and this is part of the process.

> **Considering a second opinion? Get one!** Second opinions can be sought for anything from getting more information about your diagnosis to surgical recommendations. My advice on second opinions is that if you even *think* of getting one, then get one.

There are some situations where a second opinion may not be warranted. If you have a true emergency, you probably don't have the luxury of time for another opinion. You need surgery, and you need it now. But there are also nonemergency situations where a second opinion may not be necessary. If you're confident that you understand your condition, and you know and trust your doctor, that may be all you need. I have patients I've worked with for many years. We've had a chance to establish a bond, they have confidence that the treatment we've chosen together is the right one, and some of them choose not to get a second opinion.

Some of my patients get a second opinion anyway—and I encourage them to do it. I never feel that a patient who sees another surgeon is insulting or second-guessing me, but patients are often afraid of just that. I understand not wanting to insult your doctor, but if that's how you feel about it, I've got one piece of advice: get over it. It's your back that's at risk here, and it's your interests you need to be concerned about—not your doctor's. She's an adult and she can take care of herself. If she *is* insulted by the idea of a second opinion, it's time to get a new doctor.

CHOOSING YOUR DOCTOR

Here's my cardinal rule of doctor selection: If you're uncomfortable, get a new one. So you've made the appointment, and met with the doctor, and asked some questions, and maybe even had some tests. None of that means you're obligated to stay with that doctor for the duration. If, after a couple of appointments, your doctor seems frustrated with your questions, irritated with your suggestions, or has given you reason to doubt his competence, you should go elsewhere. You are the person driving this process, and, perhaps within certain limits of geography or insurance plans, you can pick which doctor you'd like to work with. With that said, I strongly suggest that you make allowances for personal style. Not every doctor is a great communicator or has a warm bedside manner. I've known some really fine doctors with casual manners or gruff exteriors. Don't be fooled.

There is one particular scenario that I've seen play out time and time again, and it's a scenario you need to avoid. Because treating backs is an uncertain business, and there's often no surefire way to pinpoint the source of pain, it's not unusual to have an excellent doctor tell you she's not sure what's wrong with you, and have a terrible doctor tell you she is sure. It's always tempting to assume that the doctor who says she's sure is the good doctor, and vice versa, but that's often not the case.

When choosing a surgeon, remember that treatment doesn't always end after the surgery. Spinal surgery can have both short- and long-term repercussions, and the patient-surgeon relationship sometimes goes on much longer than most patients suspect. Find a surgeon you are comfortable with so if something does need further treatment, you're in good hands.

RED FLAGS

It's not easy to evaluate a doctor. I've given you some clues about what makes a good surgeon, and some sources to help you find one, but this chapter wouldn't be complete without a list of red flags that should make you seriously consider not just a second opinion but a different surgeon. If any of these sound familiar, you just might need a new doctor:

- You feel you can live with your back problem, and it's not dangerous, but he recommends surgery anyway.
- Bulging discs are the primary reason for surgery.
- You have a herniated disc, but no symptoms, and your doctor wants to operate.
- Your surgeon says, "Once I get inside, I'll see what's going on."
- Your surgeon recommends surgery without discussing alternative treatments.

- You don't know why you're having surgery.
- Your surgeon has developed a new procedure, with great results, not offered elsewhere for your condition.
- Your surgeon guarantees a cure.
- Your surgeon recommended surgery based solely on an MRI, without doing a history or a physical examination.
- Your surgeon discourages you from getting a second opinion.

CASE STUDY

BERNARD went to see a surgeon because he had numbness in his ankle. It wasn't painful, it wasn't incapacitating, and it wasn't getting worse. The surgeon determined that the source of the numbness was his spine, because Bernard had a degenerated disc that showed up on an X-ray and an MRI. The surgeon did a discogram that, in his mind, confirmed the diagnosis, and recommended that Bernard have a spinal fusion. What he didn't do was clearly explain the risks of spinal fusion versus the annoyance of living with a numb ankle. Bernard had the surgery. Not only did the fusion not cure the numbness, but Bernard ended up with chronic back pain as a result. After a year of treatment, including physical therapy, he went back to the surgeon, who said the fusion had healed properly, and that there was nothing more to be done. That's when Bernard came to see me, and I had to tell him that his surgeon was right about one thing—there was nothing more to be done.

Picking a doctor isn't easy, but if I had to boil this chapter down to one piece of advice, this would be it: Don't be afraid. Find a qualified doctor, ask questions, explore all of the alternatives, and know that you'll be able to make difficult decisions with confidence.

After you find your doctor, the most important information you can give her is a description of your symptoms. One of them may be pain. If so, the next chapter will help you to understand the type of pain you are experiencing and to describe it to your doctor.

ENDNOTE

i S. Mathur, N. Shanti, M. Brkaric, et al., "Surfing for Scoliosis: The Quality of Information Available on the Internet," *Spine* 30, no. 23 (2005), pp. 2695–2700.

THE
CAUSES OF
BACK PAIN

Chapter 4

MY BACK HURTS:
THE VARIETIES OF PAIN

Since pain is the only symptom most back problem sufferers ever have, it's important to understand it and be able to describe it. "Ouch" just doesn't cut it. If you want to treat your pain successfully, you have to make sure you know where it hurts, when it hurts, how it hurts, and how much it hurts. This may seem pretty obvious, but I see patients every day who can't go much beyond "My back hurts."

As you start to make decisions about what to do about your pain, keep in mind that it's often impossible to figure out whether the spine is the source of any particular patient's problem. Chances are good that it isn't, since most back pain is caused by something other than the spine. Even if we can determine that the spine is the problem, we may not be able to figure out just what it is about the spine that's bothering you.

Back pain isn't always spine pain. The vast majority—some 85 percent—of back pain has no known cause.[i,ii] The pain can be caused by muscles or tendons or ligaments or internal organs. It could have roots in psychosocial or emotional issues, or any one of a number of other sources.

You'll be glad to know, though, that there are situations where we can successfully diagnose back pain, and have a good shot at treating what's wrong. To understand why that's true, and to figure out if you have one of the diagnosable conditions, one of the important questions you have to be able to understand—and answer—is whether nerves are involved. If they are, there's a better chance you'll get a definite diagnosis and diagnosis-specific treatment. If they're not, treating the pain, rather than trying to find the cause, is probably the best strategy for success.

If you're thinking back to high school biology and have a hazy memory of being told that all pain comes from nerves, you may be confused. Let me clarify. When I talk about back pain with nerve involvement, I'm referring specifically to pain caused by mechanical compression of the spinal nerves; these are the ones that run through the spinal canal and out between the vertebrae. This is the kind of pain that is most likely to be treatable with surgery. You'll know how to identify it by the time you finish this chapter.

The nerves that are involved in the other kinds of low back pain are microscopic local nerves, and their activation, which you feel as back pain, generally doesn't come from something spine surgery can fix. Remember that surgery is a mechanical solution. I can relieve spinal nerve–related pain because I can physically remove whatever it is that's pressing on the nerve. In contrast, because the local nerves that branch out to muscles, tendons, facet joints, and other structures are so small—too small to be clearly visible—a mechanical solution is ineffective.

If you're just beginning to try to figure out what kind of pain you have, and what might be causing it, the most important thing you can do is pay attention. The better you can describe your pain to your doctor, the more likely it will be that you and he can treat it effectively. These are the kinds of questions you should be able to answer when you make your first appointment:

How intense is your pain?

Most doctors use a 0–10 scale, where 0 is no pain and 10 is unbearable pain.

How long have you been feeling the pain?

Months or years? Has it intensified or changed? Is it always there, or do you go for stretches without it?

Have you ever had a similar problem before?

When was it? What happened?

Where is your pain?

Is it your entire back? A well-defined area? Do you feel it in your buttock or your leg?

How would you describe the pain?

Is it dull or sharp, intermittent or constant? Is it throbbing, or does it come in twinges or spasms?

When do you feel the pain?

Is it worse at certain times of the day? When you move a certain way? After sitting still? Does it wake you up at night?

What makes it better or worse?

Does standing help? How about sitting or lying down? Walking?

Are other symptoms associated with the pain?

Numbness, tingling, weakness, burning, electrical sensations, change in bowel or bladder function?

Your doctor will also ask you about symptoms that may have nothing to do with pain. In chapter 5 we'll look at indications of a serious underlying condition, but it's worth mentioning here as well. If you have night pain, unintentional weight loss, or fevers and chills, you might have a serious infection or even cancer.

Generally, though, pain is all there is, and once you can describe your pain accurately and in detail, you'll be able to move on to the next step, which is categorizing it as involving nerves or not involving nerves. Let me first talk about two distinct kinds of pain that *don't* indicate neurological origin.

Lower back pain is localized and doesn't involve the legs, neck, or arms. This is the biggest and loosest of the categories. LBP (and you'll see that abbreviation in a lot of the literature on back pain) can be acute or chronic, intense or low-level, constant or intermittent, dull or sharp. It can be the symptom of almost any kind of back problem. You may hear LBP described as "specific" and "nonspecific." Specific LBP has a clear cause, such as a fracture, a tumor, or an infection. Nonspecific LBP is the other kind—no clear cause. About 1 percent of adults with back pain have the specific kind. Yep, 99 percent of us have the nonspecific kind, and its very lack of specificity is what makes it tricky to treat.

If you have back pain after an injury, such as a serious fall or a car accident, that pain is probably specific. Back pain that keeps getting worse, or starts to wake you up at night, may also be specific. If you have the specific kind, you need medical attention sooner rather than later. Nonspecific back pain can manifest itself in all kinds of ways. It might start up after you spent an afternoon shoveling snow or playing golf. It might be the occasional low-grade backaches you've been having ever since you can remember. Or it could be a back that starts hurting for no apparent reason whatsoever. What's most important about nonspecific pain, though, is how bad it is. Nonspecific pain may or may not need treatment, but there are no hard-and-fast rules for determining when it does. Distinguishing whether pain is specific or nonspecific isn't easy, and you need a doctor's help. Generally, the first tests your doctor does are to eliminate the specific causes of pain.

Referred pain feels like it comes from one place but actually comes from somewhere else. Kidney stones, arterial aneurysms, broken ribs, and disease of the kidney, gallbladder, and lung can all cause pain that feels like it's coming from your back. Pain from menstrual periods can also feel like back pain. That said, most back pain is back pain. Likewise, referred pain that does originate in the back can sometimes be felt in the buttocks (which my patients sometimes describe as coming from the hip). It's dull, it's achy, and it's poorly defined. We don't understand referred pain well, and it's very difficult to pinpoint its source.

And now we get to the kind of pain that does indicate neurological involvement:

Radicular pain shoots down the leg. The shooting sensation is a reliable indication that the pain comes from pressure on a nerve, and it may very well involve the spine. Few people who have back pain have radicular pain, probably less then 10 percent.

Most of my patients use "sciatica" as a synonym for radicular pain, but they're not exactly the same. "Radicular" is the generic term for pain radiating from a nerve root. The sciatic nerve runs down the back of the leg, and so radicular pain that shoots down the back of your leg may indeed be sciatica. There's also a femoral nerve, though, that runs down the front of your leg, and if that nerve is involved, you'll feel the shooting pain in front. Each of the spinal nerves that can cause pain when compressed has a particular set of symptoms and characteristic pain distribution, and I can often trace the pain precisely to its point of origin. Where you feel radicular pain can point me to exactly which nerve is being compressed.

Neurogenic claudication is pain linked to spinal stenosis. You only feel it when you are walking, not when you are standing or sitting. Some people describe it as cramping, others as throbbing. It gets worse as you walk more and stops when you stop walking and sit down. Since bending over relieves the pain, many people find relief when walking and pushing a shopping cart; the cart's handle (unlike the handle of more conventional aids, such as canes and walkers) is at just the right height to support the weight of someone bending at the waist. Patients report relief of symptoms while walking with a shopping cart so often that doctors have a name for the phenomenon—the "shopping cart sign."

All of this brings us to the all-important question: when do you see a doctor? Although I've just taken you through a long explanation of the different kinds of pain, the type you have isn't the prime determinant of whether you should pick up the phone and make an appointment. The prime determinant is simply how much it hurts. Whether it came on suddenly or gradually, whether it's sharp or dull, whether it's constant or intermittent, if the pain is bad and it doesn't seem to be improving, you should see your primary care physician. Your PCP can help you deal with a lot of different conditions that may manifest themselves in back pain, and can refer you to specialists for cases that need more attention.

Of course, if you have any of the symptoms of a serious problem that I mentioned earlier in this chapter, see a doctor immediately.

The flip side of when to see your doctor is, of course, when not to. Most back pain gets better on its own. Let's say you're otherwise healthy, and you get a sudden pain in your back after a weekend of playing golf. In that case, it's almost assuredly a problem that will resolve itself without intervention.

There are no hard-and-fast rules, and the only person who knows whether your pain is tolerable is you. If it isn't, go see the doctor.

OTHER TYPES OF PAIN

Back pain and back problems don't exist in a vacuum. My patients often have other conditions or diseases, which may or may not cause pain. Once we move beyond the back, there are many other kinds of pain, and it's important that you understand a little bit about them, if only to recognize that they're not symptoms of spine problems. They can all be serious conditions and should be treated separately from any spine-related condition.

Arthritic joint pain stemming from the hip or knee can be confused with back- and nerve-related pain. Many patients who don't know they have a worn-out hip or knee think they have a pinched nerve. A routine orthopedic evaluation and X-rays can usually uncover joint-related pain.

Neuropathic pain is pain from the nerves themselves. It isn't usually a shooting pain, which distinguishes it from radicular pain. Patients often describe it as a burning or stabbing feeling. It's often associated with numbness or other sensory disturbance. It doesn't come from a compressed nerve in the spine; it comes from a disease that affects the nerve itself. Diabetes, shingles, certain medications, and many other diseases and conditions can all cause neuropathic pain.

Complex regional pain syndrome is a problem that used to be called (among other things) reflex sympathetic dystrophy (RSD) and causalgia. It is a debilitating, localized pain in a limb that's associated with hypersensitivity and loss of function, among other symptoms. Trauma, injury, or surgery often, but not always, predates the onset of symptoms. It can be very debilitating and can go on for a very long time. Unfortunately, we don't understand it very well.

Myofascial pain has a complex definition, but the easiest way to describe it is muscle pain. It's usually characterized by localized areas of the muscle called trigger points that are tender to the touch. People with other kinds of chronic pain often have myofascial pain as well, and it sometimes lingers after other pain has subsided. Myofascial pain is suspected to be associated with other pain-causing conditions, and the best way to handle it is to treat those other conditions, as well as the pain itself.

Fibromyalgia is a syndrome that involves chronic pain as well as sleep disruption, fatigue, and mood changes. Back pain can be a component, but there doesn't seem to be a direct link to the spine.

Understanding your pain is the first step toward making the right decision about where to go from here. The kind of pain you have probably seems clear to you right now, but it's easy to lose sight of the nuances of pain types as you get into discussions of tests and abnormalities and diagnoses and treatments. As you read about all of those topics, you'll see that it always comes back to the nature and severity of what you're feeling. Pain can also be a signal of an urgent problem, or even an emergency. These are covered in the next chapter, Spine-One-One.

ENDNOTES

i American Academy of Orthopaedic Surgeons, "OKU: Orthopaedic Knowledge Update," *Spine* 3 (2006), p. 319.

ii R. A. Deyo, J. N. Weinstein, "Low Back Pain," *New England Journal of Medicine* 334 (2001), pp. 363–70.

Chapter 5

SPINE-ONE-ONE: *EMERGENCIES AND URGENCIES*

Many back problems are low-level, intermittent, or both; most don't ever rise above the level of nuisance and don't even need medical care. There are spine problems, though, that are real emergencies and require you to get to the hospital immediately. I cover them first for two reasons: because anyone who has one of them must seek treatment right away, and because anyone who doesn't can breathe a sigh of relief and get some sleep.

Most of this book is about conservative treatments. But there are cases when a patient absolutely, positively needs surgery *right now*, and the risk of postponing it far outweighs the risk of surgery. I want you to recognize the key symptoms that can indicate an emergency situation because, if you have any one of them, you should seek medical attention right away.

EMERGENCIES

My definition of an emergency is simple—it's anything that gets me out of bed at three a.m., headed straight for the emergency room. The symptoms that should set off the emergency alarm are: severe, incapacitating back or leg pain; weakness or loss of function in a limb; a sudden change in bowel or bladder control; and what's called saddle anesthesia, a loss of sensation in the genital area. The bad news is that the conditions that cause these kinds of symptoms are very dangerous; the good news is that they're very rare.

Those conditions fall into three categories:

traumatic fracture or dislocation
infections: epidural abscess and discitis
cauda equina syndrome

Traumatic Fracture or Dislocation: We'll start here because traumatic fractures are the easiest emergencies to identify. If you crash your motorcycle (you were wearing your helmet, weren't you?) or you get shot (I don't want to know . . .) and you suddenly have massive, incapacitating pain in your back, you might have a traumatic fracture. Ditto if you fall off a ladder, a horse, or a roof. Traumatic fractures aren't always quite so dramatic, though. You can fracture your spine by tripping on a curb or slipping on the ice.

There are several kinds of fractures, and all can range in severity. A *compression fracture* is when the vertebral body collapses on itself. (Trauma isn't the only cause of compression fractures. Osteoporosis can also cause them, and I describe that kind of fracture in detail in the next section.) A *burst fracture* is similar

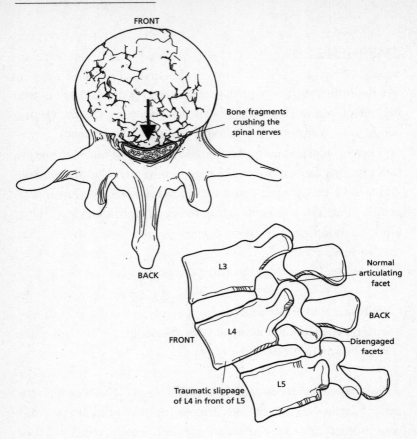

FRONT

Bone fragments
crushing the
spinal nerves

BACK

L3

Normal
articulating
facet

BACK

L4

FRONT

Disengaged
facets

Traumatic slippage
of L4 in front of L5

L5

In a burst fracture (upper left), bone fragments can compress the nerves in the spinal canal, and in a traumatic dislocation (lower right), the bones disengage from each other.

to a compression fracture, but the broken bone pushes into the spinal canal, injuring or threatening the spinal nerves. A *high-energy fracture* is a fracture caused by a lot of energy in the form of a high-speed motion or extraordinary impact. The higher the energy, the greater the damage.

Traumatic dislocations are related to traumatic fractures. They're a rare, dramatic injury where the bones in the spine actually disengage from each other—no small feat, given the way they interlock. It takes a lot of energy to do this, and you can't do it by stubbing your toe. Usually, either a fast-moving vehicle or a very serious fall is involved.

There are different ways to handle all of these injuries, but I'm not going to go into detail on them because, by the time you even know what happened, you'll be coming out of anesthesia with the fix already in. I do, however, want you to understand what they are, and how to identify a true emergency.

Symptoms: The number-one symptom of a traumatic fracture or dislocation is back pain, but there may be others. Neurological symptoms, such as numbness or tingling in the legs, loss of bowel and bladder function, and paralysis in one or both legs, can all result from a traumatic fracture. Strangely, sciatica is not a typical sign of a traumatic fracture.

Here's the bottom line: If you experience any of these symptoms after an accident—even an accident you think is trivial— you need immediate medical attention. But don't seek it under your own steam. Whatever you do, don't move. You could have an unstable spine, and moving could mean the difference between recovering and never being able to walk again. Wait until help arrives. If you happen to witness an accident, don't move the victims. Don't sit them up, and don't give them water. Call 9-1-1 and wait.

Treatments: For a severe injury, it's almost always reconstructive surgery that's called for to put things back together and realign what's been knocked out of position. For less serious fractures, a brace and time may be all that's necessary; bones, given time and stability, will heal themselves. I work in a trauma center, and I see injuries that run the severity gamut. Whether your injury is mild or severe, though, you have to focus on one thing: getting up and moving around as soon as possible after you're treated. No matter what your injury, being bed-bound only delays getting better (you'll hear me say this over and over).

Infections: In this age of antibiotics, we've gotten used to thinking of infections as something relatively minor and easily treated. When they're in the spine, though, they can be life-threatening. There are lots of nooks and crannies in your back, such as the facet joint, the epidural space, and the disc space, where infections can take hold. The bone itself can also get infected. Most spinal infections are the familiar, pus-forming kind, but tuberculosis and fungi can also infect the spine.

Infections have to come from somewhere, and one place is an invasive procedure, such as an injection, a discogram, or surgery. More commonly, an infection elsewhere in your body migrates to the spine, generally by hitching a ride in your blood. Wherever it comes from, an infection is serious. If it's in the spine, there's a risk of bone instability, nerve damage, or even paralysis. If it breaks out, it can travel to your heart, kidneys, or lungs and possibly do permanent, even fatal, damage.

Symptoms: As with other emergencies, the primary symptom is pain. At first, the pain may not be severe, but it gets worse as the infection progresses. An infection may also leave other clues. If you have fevers or chills, or have had recent unintentional weight loss, an infection might be the problem. Often, but not always, a spinal infection is preceded by an infection elsewhere in the body. Spinal infections can also (rarely) occur after invasive procedures. If the infection site is pressing on a nerve, you may also have the kinds of neurological symptoms typical of any kind of nerve compression—weakness, numbness, tingling, or bowel and bladder problems.

To determine whether your spine is infected, your doctor will probably do an MRI scan. He may also check your blood. Many infections won't show up in blood work, though, so the next step is to take a sample of the site itself.

Treatments: Sometimes antibiotics are enough. If, however, there's a collection of pus, surgery to clean up the site may be necessary. If the pus is pressing on a nerve, that surgery may be urgent. If the infection has eaten away part of a disc or bone, sometimes reconstructive surgery is required to stabilize the spine.

Cauda Equina Syndrome: If you think back (or flip back) to chapter 1, you'll remember that the cauda equina is the lower extension of the spinal cord. It's the horse's tail of nerves that's encased by the lumbar spine. Cauda equina syndrome is a massive squeezing or pinching of those nerves, and it is very, very dangerous. Even when it's properly diagnosed and treated, it can result in permanent paralysis of the legs, permanent loss of bowel or bladder function, sexual dysfunction, or numbness in the lower body.

Cauda equina syndrome is most often caused by a disc that releases a large amount of its jelly-like interior into the space through which the nerves run. The herniated material causes severe nerve compression, sometimes severe enough to permanently damage the nerve. Consequently, the bodily functions involving the nerve are also impaired. Herniation, though, is not the only cause of cauda equina syndrome. Severe spinal stenosis, burst fractures, tumors, and epidural abscesses can all cause it. Fortunately, it is not common. Don't imagine that just because you've got some sciatica you've got cauda equina syndrome.

Symptoms: There's pain, and there's nerve involvement—numbness, tingling, and weakness. There may be loss of function in the bowel or bladder, and you may either retain urine (you can't pass it) or have trouble holding it (incontinence). The genital and rectal numbness we call saddle anesthesia is also characteristic of cauda equina syndrome. Symptoms vary widely from patient to patient, and that often delays diagnosis. Once the diagnosis is made, though, it's important to get prompt treatment.

Treatments: In almost every case, surgery is the treatment for cauda equina syndrome. Whatever's pressing on the nerve has to be removed, and the only way to do that is by operating.

CASE STUDY

BRENDA is a woman in her early thirties who had given birth six months before she was seen. She'd had mild back pain during her pregnancy that resolved after delivery (which is very common). Four months later, pain came back, but a very different kind; she felt severe pain shooting down her leg. Brenda's symptoms worsened, and several weeks later she suddenly started to have difficulty holding her urine, with numbness in her genital area. She went to the emergency room, where an MRI scan revealed a large herniated disc compressing the nerves in her spinal canal. She had cauda equina syndrome, a surgical emergency.

URGENCIES

There are several conditions that, while they're not quite emergencies, do require prompt attention. I think of them as urgencies, conditions for which I'll see the patient first thing in the morning. As with most of the emergencies, the main symptom of an urgent condition is pain—severe back pain or sciatica.

But just what is severe pain? Different people define pain in different ways, and there's no objective way to measure it. It can be constant or intermittent, dull or sharp, general or localized. The simplest way to talk about it, though, is on a 0–10 scale, where 0 is no pain at all and 10 is pain you can't imagine being worse. If you're up at 9 or 10, you're definitely not reading this; you're on your way to the emergency room. If you're up around 7 or 8, you have to do something about it sooner rather than later. There's no way for you, or for me, or for anyone to know for sure that your condition is urgent, but if the pain is bad enough to make you call the doctor first thing in the morning, you may have one of the three main conditions that account for most urgencies:

acute herniated disc or low back strain

compression fracture

tumor

Acute Herniated Disc or Low Back Strain: The operative word here is "acute." Acute pain is pain that comes on all of a sudden. I'm lumping herniated disc and low back strain together because there's often no way for you, the patient, to tell them apart. There's often no way for me, the doctor, to tell them apart either. What we both know, though, is that it hurts, and we have to do something about it.

A herniated disc can be one cause of acute pain. (There is a more complete explanation of herniated discs on page 92.) There are many other causes, though—pulled muscles, inflamed tendons, and ligament injuries are just a few. "Acute low back strain" is a catchall diagnosis for anything that causes acute pain but doesn't involve spinal nerve roots.

Symptoms: Acute pain, with or without neurological involvement. If a herniated disc is the source of your pain, you might have neurological symptoms, but you might not.

Treatment: Surgery is rare, and most people get better without it. These are urgencies not primarily because there's a risk of permanent damage but because there's pain that needs to be brought under control. If there is any significant neurological involvement, such as shooting pain, weakness, or change in bowel or bladder function, then treat it as an emergency.

Compression Fractures: You already know from the Spine Tutorial in chapter 1 that vertebrae are more like eggs than stones. They have a hard outer shell called the cortical bone and softer inner material called cancellous bone (bone marrow). An osteoporotic compression fracture is when that outer shell collapses because it's been weakened by osteoporosis, and compresses the softer inner material. A comprehensive explanation of the hows and whys of osteoporosis would take a whole book. In fact, there are many good books on this topic, so I'll stick to the basics here. Osteoporosis is a condition in which essential minerals, particularly calcium, leach out of the bone. It's more common in women, but men are also susceptible.

Unless you've been tested, you don't know you have osteoporosis. It's silent and it's painless, and many of my patients only find out about it when they break a bone. (A fracture is a break in the bone—some of my patients aren't aware that those are two

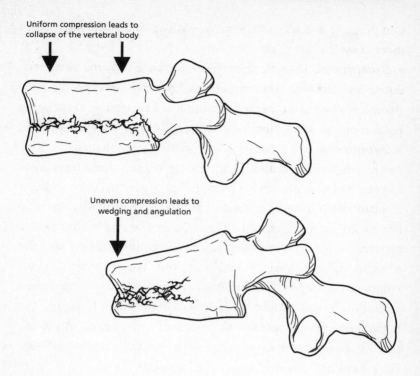

Uniform compression leads to collapse of the vertebral body

Uneven compression leads to wedging and angulation

Compression fractures happen in different ways. Some collapse evenly like a pancake (upper) and others wedge resulting in angulation or kyphosis (lower).

words for the same thing. I once told a woman with osteoporosis that she'd fractured a vertebra, and she said, with relief in her eyes, "At least I didn't break it." Now I'm quick to explain that they're synonyms.)

There are conditions other than osteoporosis that weaken bone. Cancer, kidney disease, and malnutrition can all do it. Bone is also affected by smoking, overconsumption of alcohol, inactivity, and some medications (prednisone and chemotherapeutic drugs, for example). All of these can increase the likelihood of a compression fracture, but osteoporosis is by far the most common cause.

Symptoms: There's no surefire way to know you've experienced an osteoporotic compression fracture. Some people have them and don't even know it, and others experience excruciating pain. If you're in the "excruciating pain" camp, you need prompt attention.

The single biggest risk factor for an osteoporotic fracture is having had one already, which makes sense, because fixing a fracture doesn't stop the disease. If you've already had one, you have a 20 percent chance of having a second one within twelve months.[i] If you've had two, you are even more likely to have a third. If you haven't had one, but you're elderly, post-menopausal, or you've taken medications that can compromise your bones, you might suspect a compression fracture, but there's no way to know for sure without being tested. An X-ray usually shows the fracture itself; further testing helps me figure out what kind it is, and what to do about it.

Treatments: The course of action depends on the severity of the broken bone. There are two technical measurements of severity, both of which are assessed with an X-ray (see illustration page 61). The first is simply the loss of height of the vertebral body. If it's compressed to half its pre-fracture height, it's called a 50 percent loss of height compression fracture. The other measurement is angulation. The broken vertebra doesn't always flatten like a pancake. If there's more compression in the front, the compressed vertebra looks more like a slice of pie (the technical name for this is kyphosis), and your doctor will measure the angulation in degrees.

These measurements are important, but, for me, they're not the determining factor in treatment. Pain is. I've seen fractures with as much as a 50 percent loss of height and twenty degrees of angulation that cause very little pain, as well as fractures that are much less severe but cause intense pain. If the pain indicates nerve involvement (shooting pain, numbness, tingling, loss of bowel or bladder function), that's a sign that the fracture is severe and needs to be handled right away. If the pain is limited to the back, though, it's the intensity of the pain that determines the treatment.

Treating compression fractures, particularly in the elderly, is critical. An untreated osteoporotic compression fracture can have devastating long-term consequences. While most patients heal completely and bounce back, a few develop chronic pain. Research shows that the survival rate for women aged sixty-five years or older with a vertebral fracture is lower than age-matched women without a vertebral fracture.[ii]

So what do you do? I'll start by telling you what you *don't* do. Don't stay in bed. The old-school treatment for a compression fracture was weeks of bed rest. Fortunately, we've moved on. The complications from extended bed rest range from bedsores to depression to pneumonia, and all of them disproportionately affect the elderly people who are most susceptible to compression fractures in the first place. A couple of months in bed for an elderly woman in generally poor health can lead to deterioration from which she may never recover.

Although bed rest is still part of the treatment, it's only two or three days' worth, and that's only because you may be in too much pain to move around. After those couple of days, the key to treatment is getting up and moving around. Although bending, twisting, and lifting should be avoided, walking is just about the best thing you can do. It's good for the back, but it's also good for your lungs, your heart, and your well-being, all of which play a role in recovering from any injury.

Unlike people, bones respond to stress in a good way. Bones get stronger when they're made to bear weight. While they do, though, you're probably going to be in at least some pain, and you'll need to supplement activity with some kind of pain medication.

Your doctor may also recommend one of the many different kinds of braces, but there's no clear evidence that bracing helps recovery from an osteoporotic compression fracture, and a brace may do you harm. I recommend them cautiously. (I talk about braces in some detail on page 149.)

These are all strategies to allow the fracture to heal itself. It makes sense that smaller fractures with little loss of height and little angulation heal best. Larger fractures, with more loss of height and angulation, may not heal as well. But not always. Although most fractures will heal without surgery, the height and angulation never go back to normal. The vertebra will essentially freeze in its fractured position, where it hardens and stabilizes. Sometimes, this isn't a problem. Many patients with fractures recover fully, with no pain or noticeable limitation.

When pain is unresponsive to other measures, a couple of other options come into play. They're relatively safe, minimally invasive surgical techniques with hard-to-pronounce names. Vertebroplasty and kyphoplasty are two similar procedures by which bone cement is injected into the fractured vertebra to support it from the inside while the bone heals. The key difference is that in vertebroplasty the cement is injected directly, and in kyphoplasty a balloon is first inserted into the vertebra to lift the compressed bone and make a space into which the cement can then be injected. (There's a detailed explanation of both on page 276.)

Preliminary evidence indicates that these procedures work very well for painful osteoporotic compression fractures. Patients generally see pain reduction in the 60–80 percent range, and they're up and about almost as soon as the procedure is done. Vertebroplasty has the advantage of being a simpler procedure, but the disadvantage of not significantly restoring vertebral height or repairing angulation. Kyphoplasty is a more demanding procedure for the surgeon, but it can partially restore the vertebra to its original size and shape. So far, there's no research comparing outcomes for the two.

Both of these procedures are very safe. I've done a lot of them and have had very few problems. Nevertheless, we don't know the long-term risks. Medium-term risks, though, are minimal, and the level of patient satisfaction is high. Patients who've had either procedure often come back to me for the same treatment if they have the misfortune to fracture another vertebra. It's almost unheard of for a vertebra that's been treated with one of these procedures to fracture again.

Reconstructive surgery for a vertebral compression fracture is a rare, last-ditch measure. When a fracture is very severe, unstable, or has damaged (or threatens to damage) nerves, surgery may be the only option. One of the problems, though, is that reconstructive surgery requires implants, such as screws, hooks, and rods, and osteoporotic bone is often too soft to anchor those implants in. That's why there's such a high rate of implant failure with this kind of surgery. Nevertheless, if the fracture is severe enough, the risks of not operating may exceed the risks of operating, and surgery may be called for.

Tumors: The most common kind of tumor that affects that spine is metastatic, a tumor that comes from another part of the body, usually through the blood. Metastatic tumors are usually cancerous.

Cancer may be the word that scares my patients most, and I want to emphasize that this is very, very rare. If you have no history of cancer, pain in your back is almost never a sign of the disease. Even if you have a history of cancer, it's much more likely that the pain in your back is something else. Nevertheless, it's prudent to get it checked.

The spine may occasionally play host to a nonmetastatic tumor, which could be a primary bone tumor, multiple myeloma, lymphoma, or a tumor of the spinal cord or nerves. There are many different kinds of these tumors, with subtle differences, slightly different presentations, and different treatment options. This book isn't long enough to do justice to this topic, and I'll say, one more time, that these tumors are very rare. If you are diagnosed with one, you need to see a specialist, who will tell you more than I have space for about the kind of tumor you have and what your choices are.

Symptoms: There aren't any particular symptoms indicating that you have a tumor rather than something else.

Treatments: Radiation, chemotherapy, and surgery are how tumors are treated. This is where your oncologist comes in.

If you read this chapter top to bottom, it's easy to come away with the grim idea that back pain is a sign of dangerous and even deadly problems. Although it can be, it almost always isn't. If you have back pain, you're very unlikely to find its cause in this chapter. For any given patient, the information here is much more likely to rule out a serious condition than it is to identify it. The next chapter describes many of the tests used to diagnose spinal conditions. Whether you are going to have an MRI scan or an EMG, make sure you read that chapter so that you know what to expect.

ENDNOTES

i R. Lindsay, et al., "Risk of New Vertebral Fracture in the Year Following a Fracture," *Journal of the American Medical Association* 285, no. 3 (2001), pp. 320–23.

ii D. M. Kado, et al., "Vertebral Fractures and Mortality in Older Women: A Prospective Study," *Archives of Internal Medicine* 159, no. 11 (1999), pp. 1215–20.

Chapter 6

TESTING, TESTING:
X-RAYS, SCANS, AND MORE

I f you come to me with a back problem, the most important thing I will do is take a thorough history and conduct a complete physical exam. Many people have begun to think of tests as high-tech procedures that eliminate the need for the history and physical exam. They are wrong. From hearing what it is that's bothering you and taking a good close look, I can go a long way toward identifying your problem. I believe that this remains a cornerstone of diagnosing spinal problems, and tests are adjuncts. They're very useful adjuncts, though. Although I can tell a lot by poking and prodding, I can't see your spine. Until I develop X-ray vision (Superman should have been a spine surgeon), I'm stuck doing tests that can "see" it for me.

Most patients who go to a doctor with severe back pain end up having at least one of the tests in this chapter. Some have almost all of them. But before you have a test—any test—you should understand what it is, what it can find (and not find), how risky it is, whether it's painful, and why your doctor thinks you should get it. Many of my patients have the idea that, if it's a test, it's harmless: it's only a test. The reality is that some tests are more dangerous than some surgical procedures. And they are sometimes done unnecessarily.

This chapter will acquaint you with the alphabet soup of spine tests and give you a good idea of which might, or might not, be appropriate for you. Before we get into the nitty-gritty, though, there's a word you need to know: "invasive." You've probably heard tests described as invasive or noninvasive, and I've found that many of my patients don't know what the difference is or why it's important. The difference is simply whether your perimeter is breached—by a needle through your skin or a tube down your throat or a catheter in your bladder. Literally, invasive means you're invaded. It's important because as soon as something passes into your body, the risks go up. Noninvasive tests generally have very little risk. Invasive tests can pose significant risks.

WHAT YOU NEED TO KNOW ABOUT TESTS

Most of the questions you should ask before you decide to go ahead with a test are pretty straightforward. You should know what your doctor is looking for and what the risks of the test are. You should know who is going to do the test (and, particularly in the case of invasive tests, what that person's experience is), and whether you can expect to feel pain. But there's something else, something arguably more important, that I think you have to understand before you get a test done: what the potential treatments are for the conditions you're being tested for, and how the test will affect the treatment decision.

Let me give you two examples using the same test—an MRI

scan. If you have terrible radicular pain in your leg, your doctor may suspect a herniated disc. Since one treatment may be a laminectomy to remove the disc fragment crushing your nerve, it's quite reasonable for your doctor to be testing for herniation. If he finds it on the MRI (and you meet the other criteria that make you a candidate for a laminectomy), he may recommend the procedure.

If, however, your doctor suggests an MRI scan because you have back pain and he thinks you have a degenerated disc, you need to think twice. What are you going to do if the MRI shows a degenerated disc? If you believe fusion surgery is not the answer (that is what I believe, and I hope you'll also believe it by the time you finish reading this book), then just what are you going to do with those MRI results? Try physical therapy? Exercise? Find a chiropractor? Take pain medication? Maybe all of these. But that's exactly what you'd do if you didn't get the MRI scan, so what's the point?

Even if there is no point, you may still be wondering what the harm is. An MRI scan is noninvasive, almost risk-free, and it just might turn up something.

But that *is* the problem. Chances are good that the MRI *will* turn up something (very few of us have perfect spines), and although you and your doctor may look at that something and decide to try physical therapy, exercise, and pain medication, that's not the only (or even the usual) course of action. Instead, that something that shows up on the scan could be the first step in a long series of tests, office visits, diagnoses, and treatments that will culminate in surgery. And it may turn out that that something wasn't the culprit after all. It may turn out that the something was nothing.

I've seen how that dynamic has played out and there is evidence that indicates that it's widespread. Rates of spine surgery around the country, which vary tremendously, are very telling. One region in the state of Oregon has many more surgeries per capita than another region in the state of Maine. And the same region in Oregon also has many more imaging tests than the same region in the state of Maine.[i] Coincidence? I think not. The fact that they're correlated doesn't necessarily mean that increased use of imaging tests causes increased surgery, but it's a reasonable hypothesis. Tests find abnormalities, and doctors look for a way to fix them.

That phenomenon is well enough known to have a name: the cascade effect. Here's how it's described in a paper published in 2002 in the *Annual Review of Public Health*:

Cascade effect refers to a process that proceeds in stepwise fashion from an initiating event to a seemingly inevitable conclusion. With regard to medical technology, the term refers to a chain of events initiated by an unnecessary test, an unexpected result, or patient or physician anxiety, which results in ill-advised tests or treatments that may cause avoidable adverse effects and/or morbidity.[ii]

Our poor understanding of back pain makes spinal imaging one of the areas of medicine where the cascade effect can lead to unnecessary surgery. The 2002 article specifically mentions it:

Spinal MRI exemplifies the problem of discovering more and more abnormalities with most having no clinical relevance. There are now many studies of asymptomatic patients demonstrating that herniated discs, degenerative discs, and bulging discs are frequent incidental findings. Clinically, such findings lead to overdiagnosis, anxiety on the part of the patients, and conviction about the presence of disease. Some authors have suggested that clinically irrelevant findings on MRI may lead to unnecessary back surgery.[iii]

I know it's hard to understand the idea that a very-low-risk test that gives a lot of information, such as an MRI scan, can be a bad idea. We're accustomed to thinking of the risks of tests as what can go wrong during them. With an MRI scan, though, the harm isn't in the test itself. The harm is entirely dependent on how the test is used.

> **Any test can be dangerous**—not just because it can hurt you, but because of the incidental findings it can uncover. Studies show a correlation between the number of tests obtained and the volume of surgery based on those tests, a phenomenon called the "cascade effect."

Which brings me to a reality check. I realize that it's the rare patient who will use this rationale to forgo an MRI scan. If you're in pain, both you and your doctor are probably going to want to get a good look at your spine, even if the results won't change your treatment options. It's part curiosity and part due diligence, and I understand it completely. I would never deny a patient an MRI on this basis, but I would—and I do—point out to my patients with chronic back pain that we need to treat the pain, not the abnormality on the test. (All of this, of course, assumes that we have eliminated the possibility of any urgent condition that requires treatment.)

Fortunately, simply being aware that the cascade effect exists can help you avoid it.

SEEING ISN'T KNOWING

Even if you ask all of the right questions and you're convinced that a test is valuable, you shouldn't go into it thinking that it will give you and your doctor the last word on what's wrong with you. There are many situations in which all the tests in the world don't add up to certainty. Sure, they can show me abnormalities, but they usually can't tell me what those abnormalities are doing to you. Although some tests are supposed to do that, none can do it reliably. Even if I could open up every patient and look for disc damage or stenosis or osteoporosis, I couldn't always say for sure what the problem is. Tests are clues, and they can often rule things out, but the results can also be blind alleys and red herrings, showing "problems" that aren't problems at all and telling me nothing about where the pain is really coming from.

Don't go into tests thinking they are magic, and that if you just have enough of them you'll find the answer.

Now that I've told you what tests can't do, let me tell you what they can do. Here's a synopsis:

TEST TABLE

Test	Sees	Helps Diagnose	Invasive	Advantages	Disadvantages
MRI scan	Everything • Discs • Bones • Soft tissue • Nerves	• Degenerated disc • HNP • Spinal stenosis • Fractures • Infection • Tumors	No	• Painless • Low-risk • Yields much information • No radiation	• Most likely to lead to cascade effect (although every test on this list can) • Claustrophobic • Time-consuming
X-ray	• Broken bones • Alignment • Disc space • Lesions • Implants	• Fractures • Scoliosis • Kyphosis • Degenerated discs • Bone spurs	No	• Painless • Easy • Fast • Inexpensive • Low-risk	Small exposure to ionizing radiation
CT scan	Everything an X-ray sees with better clarity	Same as X-rays but also: • Spinal stenosis • HNP • Tumors	No	• Best visibility for bones • Painless • Low-risk	Exposure to radiation
Myelogram	Nerves	• Compressed nerve • Spinal stenosis	Yes	Alternative/ adjunct to MRI	• Invasive • Exposure to contrast dye • Painful
Nuclear bone scan	New bone formation	• Fractures • Tumors • Arthritis • Infection	Yes	Highly sensitive	• Low specificity (doesn't identify a cause) • Exposure to radiation
Electro-myography	Nerve and muscle abnormalities	Nerve and muscle diseases	Yes	Helps diagnose nerve and muscle problems	• Painful • Least likely to alter treatment
Discogram	Discs	Painful disc	Yes	Controversial	• Very painful • Dubious results • Exposure to contrast dye and radiation

MAGNETIC RESONANCE IMAGING (MRI)

Magnetic resonance imaging, as the name suggests, uses giant, powerful magnets to generate an image of your spine and the nerves and soft tissues around it. It's a noninvasive test, and it's not painful or difficult, but it requires that you lie (or, in some cases, stand) still in a small space for up to an hour.

WHAT MRI SCANS CAN SEE

discs (herniated, degenerated, damaged)

bones (and whether they have lesions or infections)

soft tissue (stenosis; problems with tendons, ligaments, or muscles)

nerves (and whether they're compressed)

WHAT MRI SCANS CAN'T SEE

bone details (the severity of fractures)

details of alignment and stability (for which X-rays are clearer)

TYPES OF MRI

Open and closed machines are two formats of the machine, but they operate on the same principle. The closed machines have stronger magnets, and they give far better images. The open machines aren't as confining, but they have weaker magnets that result in lower-quality images. A magnet's strength is measured in teslas, and strong machines use magnets of 1.5 teslas, while weak machines use magnets of a fraction of a tesla.

The open machines, including the stand-up variety, exist because the closed machines are very difficult for people who are claustrophobic, and they're too small for people who are significantly overweight. If you fall into either category, your only option may be an open MRI, although sometimes claustrophobic patients can endure a closed machine with sedation.

MRI scans with contrast give detail that garden-variety MRI scans can't. If your doctor needs that detail, he'll insert a catheter into your vein and then take a scan while contrast material is fed through the catheter. The material concentrates in certain problem areas of the spine and appears on the MRI scan. Because it accumulates in different concentrations in different kinds of tissue, it helps the doctor to differentiate them. It's particularly helpful in spotting scar tissue, tumors, and infections. The use of contrast turns a noninvasive test into an invasive one, but the additional risks of injury or infection are small. There isn't a risk of allergic reaction to the contrast material, because it's not iodine-based. If you've had an allergic reaction to the contrast dye used in another kind of test, tell your doctor, but don't worry about having the same problem with an MRI scan. The contrast used in an MRI rarely causes allergy. For most purposes, though, an MRI scan without contrast suffices.

Risks: There aren't many, but you may occasionally see news stories about people who are injured (or, very rarely, even killed) when they're hit with metal objects attracted by the huge magnets in MRI machines. Virtually all MRI risks have to do with the danger of ferrous metals (those are metals that have iron in them) in the vicinity. Sometimes the metal is in objects inadvertently brought into the room, but sometimes the object is inside you. If you've got anything on this list, you *cannot* have an MRI scan:

pacemaker
mechanical heart valve
aneurysm clip
implants or cardiac stents of certain types

If there's any foreign body in your body, whether it's shrapnel or implants, make sure that you tell your doctor. It won't necessarily mean you can't have the test, but it might. If you've had fusion surgery and have any kind of instrumentation, such as screws, rods, or wires, you can usually have an MRI scan, but the metal in the instrumentation will distort the image. Stainless steel implants are particularly distorting; titanium implants are less so. The presence of implants doesn't always mean an MRI is useless, though. Your doctor may be able to tune the machine to get a good enough picture to see what he needs to see.

X-RAYS

X-rays are the workhorse test of the spine world. They're quick, easy, painless, noninvasive, and relatively inexpensive. Most spine doctors have the equipment to do them right in the office. The films are ready right away and they tell us a lot about the spine. I see very few patients who don't have an X-ray somewhere along the line.

X-rays are very good at showing bones. I can see alignment and fractures, and although I can't see discs themselves, I can see the space between the bones where the disc is, and that can tell me a lot. If one disc space is smaller than the spaces above and below, that disc may have a problem.

WHAT X-RAYS CAN SEE

broken bones (the test used for any kind of fracture)

out-of-line vertebrae (for spondylolisthesis)

alignment (for scoliosis or kyphosis)

disc space problems (for degenerated discs, bone spurs, or disc space narrowing)

lesions (tumors)

implanted hardware (for postsurgical evaluation)

WHAT X-RAYS CAN'T SEE

soft tissue (for herniated discs, stenosis, strained muscles, tendons, or ligaments)

nerves (compressed)

mild and moderate bone density loss (for osteoporosis)

Because X-rays show so much that is fundamental to the diagnosing and treating of spines, the list of reasons your doctor would order an X-ray is very, very long. It's much easier to list the situations in which an X-ray isn't necessary, because there are only two. The first is if you've had back pain for less than six weeks, and you're improving (either with or without treatment). The second is if you've had an MRI and more information about your bones isn't necessary.

X-RAY TYPES

Digital X-rays are just normal X-rays processed by computer. It's exactly like the difference between a digital camera and a traditional film camera. Digital X-rays have the advantage of not using film.

Flexion and extension X-rays capture images of your spine bending first one way and then the other, so the doctor can compare the two to see your range of motion. For the flexion

X-ray, you'll bend forward and push your back up like a cat, then for the extension X-ray you'll lean back like you're doing a tennis serve. They are used to help determine if your spine is unstable.

Risks: The only risk of X-rays is a small exposure to ionizing radiation, but over the last couple of decades we've gotten a lot better at reducing that risk. We have better equipment, more sensitive film, and special grids that focus the radiation, and these all help minimize exposure. We use lead aprons to cover any sensitive areas of the body, such as the genitals, the breasts, and the thyroid. There is very little risk involved in X-rays. Radiation can, however, harm a fetus, so make sure to tell your doctor if there's any chance you could be pregnant.

If the idea of ionizing radiation still scares you, you should know that it's all around you. A coast-to-coast flight exposes you to a similar amount of radiation as a routine chest X-ray.

COMPUTERIZED TOMOGRAPHY (CT) SCAN

A CT scan is nothing more than a supersophisticated X-ray. Instead of a head-on view, the CT scan gives you a cross-section, with much more detail. While a CT scan doesn't show soft tissues in the spine well (nerve, disc, ligaments), it is often used as a first step for patients who can't have an MRI scan.

There are several reasons to get a CT scan. If your doctor needs a better picture of a fracture, or a closer look at a lesion, or an evaluation of the bone before doing surgery that requires screws to be implanted, he may order one. CT scans are also used to help diagnose spinal stenosis and are sometimes used in conjunction with myelograms and discograms.

CT scans are done in tunnels similar to those in MRI machines, but bigger (so claustrophobia isn't usually a problem). The test only takes a few minutes. As with X-rays, the only risk of a CT scan is radiation exposure. CT scans use more radiation than X-rays, but not enough to pose a real risk (except to pregnant women, who shouldn't have CT scans).

MYELOGRAM

All of the tests I've mentioned so far are low-risk, noninvasive procedures. A myelogram is neither. It's a test in which contrast dye is injected directly into the spinal canal, inside the lining of the nerves (called the dura). It works its way up and down the length of the spinal column (with a little help from a table that tilts you back and forth) and an inch or so down each nerve that exits the spinal canal. Once the dye is in, the nerves can be seen on X-rays and CT scans, as can anything compressing the nerves.

Myelograms were developed decades before MRI scans, and have largely been replaced by them. If you can have an MRI, it's safer to get an MRI than a myelogram. If you can't have an MRI, you may need to start with a myelogram. There are also situations in which an MRI doesn't provide enough information and a myelogram can help. Patients who have had prior surgery, especially with implants or suspected scar tissue, can benefit from a myelogram. Tumors and lesions inside the spinal canal may also be visualized with a myelogram.

Risks: Complications can be serious, but they don't happen often. While headaches are the most common side effect, inserting a needle into the spinal canal can cause much more serious problems, such as infections and leaks of spinal fluid. This kind of infection is particularly dangerous because the spinal column is the highway to your brain, and if the infection spreads you could end up with meningitis. There's also the risk of an allergy to the contrast dye.

NUCLEAR BONE SCAN

There are several different types of nuclear scans. They all involve injecting you with a radioactive substance, which collects in areas where there is something abnormal going on. By taking images of where that substance collects, we can diagnose certain kinds of conditions.

In the case of a nuclear bone scan, you get the radioactive substance (technetium-labeled phosphonates, if you want the details) injected into a vein and, after a short wait, you lie on a table that picks up radiation. The substance collects in areas of active bone formation, which could be from a fracture, infection, or tumor, because all of these spur new bone growth. Unfortunately, it can't distinguish among them. Once an abnormal area is picked up by a bone scan, another test, such as an X-ray or an MRI scan, may be necessary to make a diagnosis.

Don't confuse a nuclear bone scan with an osteoporosis scan. A nuclear bone scan looks for abnormal new bone formation, and an osteoporosis scan checks bone density. Osteoporotic bone doesn't look any different from healthy bone on a nuclear scan.

Risks: Getting injected with radioactivity sounds a lot riskier than it is. Although nuclear bone scans are invasive (because you're injected with dye), they're quite safe. There's almost no possibility of an allergic reaction to the dye because it doesn't contain iodine. There is exposure to radiation, however. As with procedures that involve radiation, if you are pregnant, or there is any chance you might be, hold off on the bone scan.

ELECTROMYOGRAPHY (EMG)

The purpose of an EMG, usually done by a neurologist or a physiatrist, is to identify a damaged or compressed nerve and find out if the muscles it leads to are affected. The problem is that this difficult, painful test diagnoses, unreliably, nerve involvement that your doctor should be able to reliably diagnose with a good physical exam, a thorough patient history, and an MRI scan. When someone comes to my office with pain, it is not difficult to determine whether there is nerve involvement. Once I know that, the next question is whether there's nerve compression in the spine, and where it's coming from. The vast majority of the time, that's pretty easy. An MRI scan will almost always tell me whether there's compression, and where that compression is.

Outside the spine field, EMGs are very useful. They can help diagnose carpal tunnel syndrome, traumatic nerve injury, and a variety of muscle- and nerve-related diseases. For back pain, their value is questionable.

EMG is shorthand for a test that has two components. The nerve conduction study (NCS) is supposed to determine whether there's nerve damage, and it's followed by an electromyography study (that's the EMG, but it is also called the Needle Electrode

Examination), which is supposed to determine whether the muscle is affected.

The NCS measures the strength and speed of impulse conduction inside the nerve. We know how fast and how strong impulses are supposed to be, and the theory is that if your impulse is too weak or too slow, there's damage to the nerve. To see whether the damage is affecting the muscle, the doctor administering the test sticks a needle in the muscle and measures its electrical activity.

So far, there is only one prospective, rigorous study of EMG involving the lumbar spine, and its conclusion is that the NCS/EMG combo can help support a diagnosis of spinal stenosis. By "support" I mean that it helps eliminate other possible diagnoses that could be confused with stenosis (such as a nerve or muscle problem unrelated to the narrowing of the spinal canal).[iv] The problem is that stenosis is one of the most straightforward spine conditions to diagnose. So having a painful, time-consuming test to verify that kind of diagnosis is close to useless. And that's the central problem with EMGs—they don't change the treatment plan.

Besides pain and uselessness, though, EMGs have other problems. Because nerve response tends to slow down as we age, it gets harder and harder to see clearly what an abnormally slow response is. For patients older than about sixty, an EMG is much more difficult to interpret.[v] Another problem is that the test is often done at the wrong time. When there's nerve damage in the back, it takes about three weeks before that damage is reflected in the muscle. On the other end of the spectrum, if you've had radicular pain for over 12 to 18 months, the test can be unreliable.[vi] Getting an EMG in the initial three weeks, or after a year or so, has diminishing results, but I've seen it happen over and over.

Another problem is how EMGs are prescribed: many doctors do it again and again. If one's good, three must be better. So it's not enough you have to undergo a painful test with iffy results once. You may be told to come back in three months to have it done again. My advice? Run away.

Do you really need an EMG? If all you have is low back pain and no neurological signs or symptoms, there is no reason to have an EMG. If you are thinking about an EMG for back-related pain, be sure to ask your doctor how the results will change your treatment. If it won't change your treatment, think twice.

If I haven't talked you out of an EMG already, you should also know that if you're on blood thinners, have a bleeding disorder or you have a pacemaker, you may not be able to have this test.

Although I think an EMG is almost never appropriate for isolated back pain, the ideal patient for it would be one who has had nerve- or muscle-related symptoms for less than a year unexplained by other tests. If that's not you, then the only reason to get an EMG is if you have more than one disease with neurological involvement. In that case, an EMG might help determine which disease is causing which symptom. Patients with both diabetes and spinal stenosis, for example, may have nerve-related symptoms from either disease, and an EMG might be able to identify the culprit.

I believe that the EMG is the most overprescribed invasive test in my field. I have patients who've had an EMG and vow they'll never have another.

DISCOGRAM

As a test, the discogram is in a class by itself. Not only is there widespread disagreement about how the results of discograms should be used in diagnosis, there's even controversy over whether they measure anything at all. This sets them apart from all the tests you've read about so far. While doctors disagree about what to do about a herniated disc that shows up on an MRI scan, nobody disagrees that MRI scans show herniated discs. With discograms, doctors disagree, both about what the test measures and what to do about it.

Discograms get us into the very murky area of discogenic low back pain—pain in your lower back that seems to be coming from a disc. In general, the way doctors decide that pain seems to be coming from a disc is by a process of elimination. If the pain doesn't seem to be coming from anywhere else, then it's discogenic. Discogram proponents say the test can actually determine if the disc is the source of the pain. Discogram opponents—and I'm one—don't believe that's true.

But before we delve into whether a discogram works, let me tell you what a discogram is. It's an invasive test in which a very long needle is inserted through your back, through your spine, and directly into a disc. Contrast dye is then injected under pressure into the disc. The doctor is trying to find out if the disc hurts and if the pain you experience during the test, both in location and intensity, is the same kind of pain that drove you to go to the doctor in the first place. If it is, the doctor classifies the pain as concordant, and concludes that the disc is causing the pain. If you have no pain, or the pain feels different from your normal back pain, the theory is that the disc is probably not causing it.

Your doctor will also evaluate the way the dye distributes itself in your disc. During or directly after your test, your doctor will take X-rays (and likely CT scans) of the test site. In a normal disc, the dye collects in the soft inner core, and looks like a marshmallow sitting between two vertebrae on the X-rays. If the disc is damaged or degenerated, the dye will escape from the center and be visible around the periphery of the disc. The disc will also take more dye before it's filled up (a natural consequence of some of the dye escaping the center). The point of this analysis is to figure out whether the disc is damaged. If it is damaged, that's one more piece of information to help conclude that it's causing pain. If it's not damaged, but you have concordant pain, many doctors will still conclude that the disc is the problem and use the discogram result to consider surgery.

I have a couple of problems with conclusions based on discogram results. First, if you inject enough dye under enough pressure into any disc, you can make any patient scream in pain. (I've heard the test referred to as a screamogram.) Second, it doesn't seem completely rational to me to believe that by injecting a disc with dye you can conclude that the disc is painful under everyday conditions. As you go about your life, there are no circumstances under which dye is injected into your discs. So why, just because it hurts when *that* happens, should we conclude that your everyday pain is in any way related?

One interesting study looked at discogram results in a group of people who didn't have back pain (I'm not sure how they convinced people to participate in *that* one). Some had pain during the test; others didn't. They were all followed for four years, and it turned out that the ones with "positive" discograms weren't any more likely to develop back pain than those with "negative" test results.[vii] That's not conclusive evidence that discograms don't tell you anything, but it's not an endorsement of the test, either.

If you're determined to have a discogram, though, I have a piece of advice: Get one from someone other than your surgeon, or any doctor who knows which disc is suspect. The test should be done "blind" by a doctor not involved in your care. Your surgeon should instruct him to test at least two discs—the target disc and one other—without knowing which is suspected (and don't tell him). Because the results of a discogram are seldom clear, and they require interpretation, having a different doctor perform the test and interpret the results reduces the chance that your doctor will simply confirm his own beliefs. (For the same reason, you shouldn't know which discs are being tested.) Many surgeons prescribe the test this way, for this reason.

The North American Spine Society, which is the largest society of physicians treating the spine in the world, has specific guidelines for the use of the discogram.[viii] If you are going to have a discogram, discuss those guidelines with your surgeon and be sure that your condition falls within them.

Discogram Bottom Line: Unless you are committed to having a spinal fusion (or disc replacement), there is no reason to consider this controversial, painful, and invasive diagnostic-only procedure.

WHY A DISCOGRAM?

The only purpose of a discogram is to verify that a disc is causing pain. It can't diagnose a herniated disc, spinal stenosis, spondylolisthesis, fracture, infection, tumor, or anything else. And even if you believe that discograms can do what they're supposed to do—reliably pinpoint a painful disc—there's only one reason to get one: you're considering surgery for that disc. If you'd prefer to try alternatives to surgery, the discogram will tell you absolutely nothing that will change your choice of treatments.

The natural question, then, is whether surgery works any better for patients who have had a "positive" discogram than for patients who've had no discogram; we don't know the answer. Until we do, in the words of a review of research studies involving the test, "it is not possible to endorse or deny the value of [a discogram] to surgical outcomes."[ix] Some doctors justify doing the test by arguing that a negative discogram is a good reason not to get surgery, but I know a lot of good reasons not to get surgery that don't involve needles, risks, pain, and controversy.

Even though discograms have been around for forty years, and we have no other test that is supposed to identify a painful disc, many doctors believe the results can be misleading.

Risks: There are some risks inherent in the procedure, and the possible complications include infection, injury to structures around the injection site, allergic reaction to the dye, and spinal fluid leaks. Beyond that, we don't know whether there are long-term consequences to injecting dye into a disc. The biggest risk, though, is the risk of a false positive. Positive discogram results may lead your surgeon to recommend fusion surgery. If those results are wrong, you've just had major, risky surgery for no reason.

Now that you know all about tests, it's time to find out about the kinds of problems they help diagnose, with their characteristic symptoms and treatment options.

ENDNOTES

i J. D. Lurie, N. J. Birkmeyer, J. N. Weinstein, "Rates of Advanced Spinal Imaging and Spine Surgery," *Spine* 28, no. 6 (2003), pp. 616–20.

ii R. A. Deyo, "Cascade Effects of Medical Technology," *Annual Review of Public Health* 23 (2002), pp. 23–44.

iii Ibid.

iv A. J. Haig, et al., "The Sensitivity and Specificity of Electrodiagnostic Testing for the Clinical Syndrome of Lumbar Spinal Stenosis," *Spine* 30, no. 23 (2005), pp. 2667–76.

v K. R. Chemali, B. Tsao, "Electrodiagnostic Testing of Nerves and Muscles: When, Why, and How to Order," *Cleveland Clinic Journal of Medicine* 72 (2005), pp. 37–48.

vi Ibid.

vii E. Carragee, et al., "Prospective Controlled Study of the Development of Lower Back Pain in Previously Asymptomatic Subjects Undergoing Experimental Discography," *Spine* 29, no. 10 (2004), pp. 1112–17.

viii R. D. Guyer, D. D. Ohnmeiss, A. Vaccaro, "Lumbar Discography," *The Spine Journal* 3, no. 3S (2003), pp. 11s–27s.

ix Ibid.

Chapter 7

THE USUAL SUSPECTS: *COMMON BACK DIAGNOSES*

The spine is complicated. It has many different functions, all of which are essential to living a normal life, and lots of moving parts, any one of which can fail. If you're reading this book, you probably have an idea that one of yours has failed. You may even already have a diagnosis. This chapter is where you'll find a comprehensive and comprehensible explanation of just what that diagnosis means. It will also begin to answer that all-important question: to operate or not to operate?

Before I get to the individual diagnoses, there's one point I'd like to get across. Every day I see patients who have been diagnosed with one thing or another, and I've found that "diagnosis" is a big, important word to most of them. It means that something's wrong, that we know what it is, and that treatment is necessary. In reality, though, none of those things may be true.

It is very tempting to draw a bright line between normal and abnormal, where normal means perfect and abnormal means imperfect. If that were our working definition, though, we'd define normal almost out of existence; very few of us have perfect spines. Many of us have a bone spur (diagnosis: degenerative disc disease), a leaky disc or two (diagnosis: herniated disc), or a dark area that shows up on an MRI scan (diagnosis: black disc), and live perfectly normal lives.

> **Focus on your pain, not your diagnosis.** In most cases of back pain, what determines whether you need treatment is not your diagnosis but the severity of the pain.

Once your doctor has ruled out a serious cause for your back pain, figuring out whether you have a degenerated disc, a bone spur, or an arthritic facet is not as important as treating the pain itself. I don't usually measure the severity of the problem by the extent of the physical abnormality I see on a test result. The degree to which your disc is degenerated matters much less to me than the intensity of your pain.

A diagnosis is important because it gives me some clues to treating your pain, but, by itself, it doesn't tell me where on the severity continuum you are. Every diagnosis I cover here can be either trivial or serious, and you shouldn't make the mistake of thinking that just because you have a piece of paper with one of these diagnoses written on it, you need to consider surgery.

Some people have conditions that are straightforward to diagnose, for which surgery is clearly indicated and generally successful. A small percentage of people with back pain fit into this group. Those people are the ones whose lives are immeasurably improved by surgery, but they're also the ones who give misplaced hope to the less fortunate patients whose problems don't lend themselves to surgical solutions.

The diagnoses covered in this chapter are:

- herniated disc: leaking of disc material into the spinal canal
- spinal stenosis: narrowing of the spinal canal
- spondylolysis: fracture in a part of the vertebra
- spondylolisthesis: an out-of-line vertebra
- kyphosis: loss of the normal swayback in the lumbar spine
- facet joint syndrome: degeneration of the joints holding the vertebrae together
- scoliosis: abnormal lateral curvature of the spine
- sacroiliac joint problems: degeneration of the joint that connects the sacrum to the pelvic bone
- discogenic low back pain: any kind of pain attributed to a disc, including:
  □ degenerative disc disease and black disc
  □ internal disc disruption
- acute low back pain

HERNIATED DISC

The name of this condition has led to a lot of misunderstanding. "Herniated" means moved out of its normal position. Most of us know it from the very accurately described "hernia," which is when intestines pop out of the abdominal cavity. You'd think, from the name, that a herniated disc slips out of place (especially since one of its aliases is "slipped disc"), but that's not what happens.

Remember that a disc is like a jelly donut, with a soft material (the nucleus) surrounded by firmer material (the annulus). When you move, bend, and lift, you put pressure on your spine and the disc acts as a shock absorber. But if you've ever bitten into a donut a little too aggressively and ended up with raspberry jam down your shirt, you can picture what happens to a disc that can't take the pressure. We don't have a good idea of why some discs spring a leak while others seem to take the same amount of pressure without herniating, but leaky discs are very common.

The same concept covers a lot of slightly different diagnoses. Leaky discs are also known as slipped, prolapsed, extruded, sequestered, displaced, ruptured, or protruded. (Note that "bulging" disc isn't on the list. It's a different condition, and I'll cover it in a moment.) The names all refer to the degree to which the disc leaks. In some cases only a little bit of nucleus leaks out (protruded), and in others more nucleus comes out (extruded). In extreme situations, enough nucleus drips out that it separates

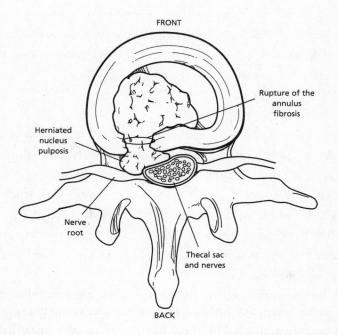

Top down view showing a herniated disc compressing the exiting spinal nerve and other nerves inside the thecal sac.

from the disc of origin (sequestered). The bigger the leak, the greater the chance of nerve compression. All of these can also be called "displaced," for the simple reason that they all involve material that's not where it's supposed to be.

Although there are official standards for these terms (I took the liberty of simplifying them a bit), doctors don't always interpret the same disc the same way.[i] One surgeon's protruded disc may be another's extruded disc, and there's no referee to call the play. The important question, though, isn't what to call it, but what to do about it. The danger of a herniated disc is that the escaped nucleus can press on a nerve.

> **When it comes to a herniated disc, size does matter.** The smaller the herniation, the less likely it is to cause nerve-related problems and respond to surgery.

A bulging disc hasn't leaked and is therefore not herniated. "Bulging" simply means that the contour of the disc is not perfect, and it's not a diagnosis. It's just a description. And most of us have at least one disc that fits that description. One study that looked at people with no back pain whatsoever found that over half of them had at least one bulging disc;[ii] other studies showed similar findings. And the older you are, the more likely it is that some of your discs bulge.

A recent task force of three spine societies addressed the bulging disc issue in a 2001 article: "The term 'bulging disc' has been used to mean many things and has caused a great deal of confusion. . . . Its use as a general term to signify disc displacement should be avoided. . . . Bulging, by definition, is not a herniation. . . . Application of the term 'bulging' to a disc does not imply any knowledge of etiology, prognosis, or need for treatment or necessarily imply the presence of symptoms."[iii] Bulging discs are an everyday finding, and there's no evidence that they cause pain. I don't think you have to do anything about them.

> **If you have a bulging disc, rest easy—you don't have a herniated disc.** In fact, you don't even have a specific diagnosis. "Bulging" is just a radiological description of the contour of the disc. It does not indicate whether the disc is degenerated, injured, damaged, or even causes pain. No term in spine parlance has caused more confusion and led to more unnecessary treatment.

There's no incontrovertible evidence that even herniated discs cause back pain. MRI scans of people with no back pain frequently show a herniation somewhere along the spine. The numbers are high: If you're under sixty, and pain-free, there's a 20 percent chance your scan will find a herniation; if you're past sixty, the chance goes up to 36 percent.[iv] The same task force that described bulging discs also looked at herniated discs. They concluded: "The term herniated disc does not infer knowledge of cause, relation to injury or activity, concordance with symptoms, or need for treatment."[v]

Herniated discs can cause radicular pain and can do this in one of two ways. The first is by compressing a nerve mechanically—by physically pressing on it. The second is by producing chemicals that can also irritate the nerve and send pain shooting down your leg. How much of sciatica is physical pressure and how much is chemical irritation is under investigation, but the fact that part of it is chemical may be the reason a lot of sciatica from herniated discs goes away all by itself, even when the nerve is still being compressed. The chemicals aren't the only thing that subside. The herniated portion of the disc can, over several years, be reabsorbed by the body.[vi] Aren't bodies amazing?

There's one kind of herniation that has no chance of impinging on the nerve. It's called a Schmorl's node, and it's a disc that herniates into the end plate of the vertebral body above or below. Under no circumstances should you take any action on a Schmorl's node. It won't cause pain or problems, and you can safely leave it alone. I've seen Schmorl's nodes mistaken for fractures, and my patients were very relieved to find out that they had something common and benign.

As you read through this book, you'll learn that there are all kinds of conditions that I think you should just leave alone. Try to manage the pain, and let your body do its work. If our bodies weren't marvelously adept at repairing themselves, we would have died out as a species a long time ago. It's very surprising how many problems just go away. Even something as concrete and identifiable as a herniated disc that's causing you pain today may not be a problem next week, or next month, or next year.

Symptoms: As usual, the symptom is pain, but the kind of pain is very important. A herniated disc can cause radicular pain to shoot down your leg if the herniation is in the epidural space and presses on the nerves in the spinal column. If your pain is localized in the back, or back and buttocks, it's much harder to peg it back to a herniated disc, and there's some question as to whether a herniated disc causes back pain at all. Many people with herniated discs have back pain, but many other people with herniated discs have none.

CASE STUDY

MELINDA is an endurance cyclist who came to see me with what she'd been told was hamstring tendonitis. She'd been sidelined for months by doctors who'd prescribed anti-inflammatories and physical therapy; they'd assumed that she had tendonitis because she was an athlete. She hadn't improved, and was getting depressed. A mutual friend who heard her story and suspected that tendonitis wasn't her problem sent her to me. Just hearing her describe the pain, I suspected that our friend was right. Tendonitis can mimic sciatica, but there are a couple of important differences. If the pain extends beyond the tendon, it's not tendonitis. If the tendon isn't painful to touch, it's not tendonitis. Melinda had pain all the way to her ankle, and no pain to the touch. I did an MRI and found a massively herniated disc. I performed a lumbar laminectomy, and six weeks later she was back on the bike for the first time in almost a year.

Treatment options: When there is compelling evidence that the herniated material is pressing on a nerve, and it is symptomatic, a laminectomy (the surgery is described in chapter 12) may be appropriate. The first hint that this might be the case is a symptom of nerve compression: radicular pain; numbness, tingling, or weakness in the leg or foot; or a change in bowel or bladder function. There's one particular kind of herniation that is removed without a laminectomy. If the hernia is on the far side of the disc, away from the rest of the bones and spinal column, there's no need to cut off the lamina to reach it. It's called a far lateral disc herniation, and it's rare. It can be removed without taking off the lamina because of its unique position.

If your diagnosis is a herniated disc, and your symptom is primarily or exclusively back pain (as opposed to leg pain), the odds that you'll get better with surgery are slim. In that case, my advice is to forget about the herniated disc and concentrate on treating the pain. In addition, if you do have sciatica, take heart: the odds are it will go away on its own; most patients with sciatica get better without surgery.

SPINAL STENOSIS

Spinal stenosis is the narrowing of the tube inside your spine that houses your spinal cord and nerves. That tube is called the spinal canal, and if you think of it as a garden hose, you can understand stenosis as what happens when your toddler steps on the hose when you're watering the lawn. The hose gets squashed, and the water supply gets cut. As with the toddler on the hose, there are degrees of stenosis. If the hose is barely compressed, you won't even notice the change in water flow. If more pressure is applied, you'll see the stream turn to a trickle. Enough pressure, and the water stops flowing altogether.

Most people who have spinal stenosis will never know. The narrowing is mild enough that it doesn't compress the nerves. If there is no compression, there is no problem. Even if there is compression, you may not know. You'll only know that you have stenosis—and it only becomes a problem—when you experience nerve-related symptoms.

The point at which that happens varies from person to person. One of the factors that helps determine whether stenosis compresses a nerve is the size of the spinal canal. Some people have a larger canal; other people have a smaller one. If you have a small

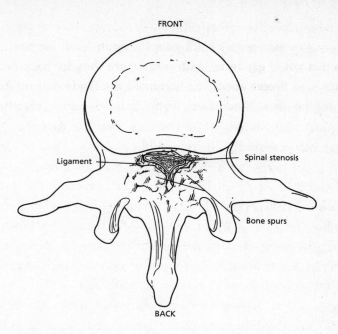

FRONT

Ligament

Spinal stenosis

Bone spurs

BACK

Spinal stenosis causes this severely narrowed spinal canal to compress the spinal nerves as they pass through the constricted area.

canal, your nerves don't have a lot of leeway. If you've got a wide canal, you've got a lot of room for stenosis.

Stenosis usually carries one of three labels that describe where in the spinal canal the impingement is occurring. Central stenosis is what it sounds like—the impingement is right in the middle of the canal, where there is normally a lot of room between nerve and bone. Two other kinds, lateral recess and foraminal, are more peripheral. Lateral recess is encroachment on the side of the spinal canal. Foraminal is encroachment not in the spinal canal itself but in the space the nerve runs through as it leaves the spinal column. It's called the neural foramen, and it's kind of an off-ramp from the spinal column. Between each two vertebrae, two nerves exit the spinal column at each level, one on either side. It is these nerves that allow your feet, or your toes, or your bladder, to communicate with your brain. Foraminal stenosis is impingement of the off-ramp rather than the highway itself.

Spinal stenosis describes anything that narrows the spinal canal and potentially puts pressure on a nerve. You've already read about herniated discs, which are their own diagnosis, but are also a cause of spinal stenosis. The most common type of stenosis is degenerative. It comes from ordinary wear and tear, combined with any one of a variety of arthritic conditions that can cause bone spurs, or pressure from loose ligaments or disc material. There are also rare kinds of stenosis, such as developmental stenosis, that can be seen in childhood.

It is rare for stenosis to be dangerous. Massively herniated discs, blood or hematoma in the spinal canal, an abscess, a tumor, or bone fragments from broken bone are causes of stenosis, and are covered in chapter 5 because they're emergencies. They can cause rapid deterioration and, possibly, paralysis, and they need immediate attention. Most stenosis, though, is much less threatening, and the kind of treatment you seek, and the speed with which you seek it, will depend on the severity of your pain.

Symptoms: The most common symptom is pain, although it can be accompanied by fatigue, heaviness in the legs, numbness, tingling, and even bowel and bladder problems. As with a herniated disc, the type of pain is critical. Degenerative spinal stenosis causes a very specific kind of pain called neurogenic claudication. "Claudication" comes from the Latin word for limping, and "neurogenic" means the problem originates in the nerves. Whoever named it could just as well have called it nerve limp, but I guess that would have made it sound too mundane. In reality, it's not mundane at all. It causes severe pain and cramping in the legs while walking, and it can be crippling. I routinely see patients whose pain is so severe, they have trouble walking to the end of the driveway to get the mail. But I also see spinal stenosis patients with only mild leg pain, or none at all. As with herniated discs, if you have only back pain, don't expect surgery for stenosis to improve it. The only kind of pain that can be reliably linked to stenosis is neurogenic.

Because neurogenic claudication is a specific, easily identifiable problem, it makes diagnosing spinal stenosis, and deciding what to do about it, relatively straightforward. You can certainly have spinal stenosis without neurogenic claudication, but then there's no need for surgery.

There is one imposter that is sometimes mistaken for neurogenic claudication: vascular claudication. If you've already guessed that it's a limp that has something to do with the blood, you're right. It's when the blood supply to your legs is constricted, generally from hardening of the arteries. Like its neurogenic cousin, vascular claudication causes pain in the legs. There are two ways to tell them apart. The first is by checking for blood flow in the leg; if you don't have a pulse in your feet, it's more likely to be vascular than neurogenic. The second is by bending over: if your claudication is neurogenic, bending your spine as you walk relieves the pain; if it's vascular, bending makes no difference. Patients with neurogenic claudication are comfortable riding a bicycle, walking uphill, or walking while leaning on a shopping cart, because all those activities are done with a bent spine. Patients with vascular claudication are not. Just to make it more difficult, it's possible for one patient to have both conditions, and they have to be treated separately.

Treatment options: As with herniated discs, the treatment depends on whether any nerves are being compromised. Even severe stenosis can be completely benign, with no symptoms and no treatment required, or life-threatening, with excruciating pain and the danger of paralysis. If your pain is severe and you are having difficulty walking, you should consider a laminectomy. If it's manageable, manage it.

SPONDYLOLYSIS

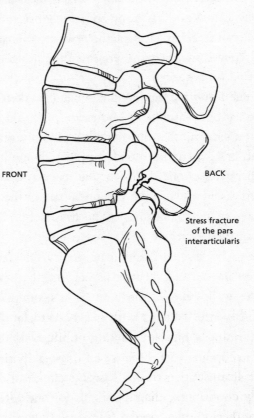

FRONT

BACK

Stress fracture of the pars interarticularis

A stress fracture, or spondylolysis, most often occurs at the pars interarticularis, as shown.

Spondylolysis is a type of stress fracture, which means that it's a fracture that comes from something other than trauma. The constant repetition of standing, sitting, bending, lifting, throwing, running, and jumping can break a bone. Shins, feet, pelvis, and hips are where stress fractures usually show up, but they can also hit the vertebrae.

Spondylolysis is a fracture of the pars interarticularis, which is a part of the vertebra that's the bridge between the two facets. Nobody knows how you get it, and we often see it in children and young adults. About 5 percent of five-to-seven-year-olds have it, and the number inches up to 6 percent by age eighteen.[vii] It hasn't been found at birth, so we know it happens during development. We often find out about it when kids start becoming physically active, because moving around, bending and stretching, can sometimes be painful. Spondylolysis is more likely to be painful when participating in sports, specifically gymnastics and football. There is limited evidence that participating in these sports increases the odds that a child will get a stress fracture, but nonathletic adolescents also have spondylolysis, and some may not even be aware of it.

Adults also have spondylolysis. We don't have a good idea of how common it is, because, although there may be lots of people walking around with it, they don't have symptoms. We find out adults have spondylolysis only if they show up at the doctor's office in pain, and tests show a fracture or spondylolisthesis (see next page).

Sometimes I can see the stress fracture on an X-ray, but X-rays can't reliably confirm the diagnosis; if I don't see it, it doesn't mean it's not there. I often need a CT scan, a nuclear bone scan or an MRI to visualize the damaged bone. Some fractures will show up on CT scans, but not bone scans, and some vice versa.

Sometimes the first two tests won't show the break, but the third test is the charm.

Symptoms: As always, it's pain: back pain, with no nerve involvement. The pain is worse with activity that involves arching your back backward, such as serving in tennis or volleyball, which puts stress on the broken bone. Gymnasts and football players are more likely to have pain due to the nature of their sports.

Treatment options: If it doesn't hurt, you don't do anything. If it hurts a lot, you treat it. The first line of treatment is modification of activity, with NSAIDs to control the pain. Physical therapy can also help. Short-term bracing is controversial but can also help, although I discourage long-term use (see page 149).

In extreme situations, surgery is warranted to fuse the bones above and below the fracture. If severe pain persists for more than six months to one year, and doesn't respond to more conservative treatments, you may need a spinal fusion. Most fusions for spondylolysis fuse the fractured vertebra to its nearest neighbor. Some surgeons, though, do what's called a direct pars repair, which essentially glues the two sides of the fractured bone together with a bone graft and wires or screws. It's a lot like fixing a crack in a plate, where you put the glue in the crack and clamp the two sides together while it sets. The studies to date on this procedure have been small, but it may be as effective as fusion.

SPONDYLOLISTHESIS

If you stand up and run your hand down the bottom part of your spine, you can feel that it curves in toward your body. You may know that as a swayback, but the technical term is "lordosis." Because your spine isn't straight up and down like an elevator shaft, the pressure on your vertebrae isn't even. There is more pressure on the inward part of the curve (which is the side of your spine closest to your back). Because of that curve, your lumbar vertebrae *want* to slip forward. It's physics. They're being pushed.

Normally, your vertebrae can withstand the pressure, but damage to the bone or facet joints can render them more susceptible to being pushed out of line. Spondylolisthesis is an out-of-line vertebra, and it's fairly common.

There are six kinds of spondylolisthesis. The first two occur during childhood and the last four occur primarily in adults.

Isthmic: This is caused by an unhealed spondylolysis. The lion's share of childhood spondylolisthesis is isthmic.

Dysplastic: This is a result of a longer-than-normal pars interarticularis. When that part of the vertebra is elongated, it pushes the base of the bone out of line with the rest of the spine. It primarily affects the lowest lumbar vertebra, and results in a slip between the L5 and S1 vertebrae. Close to 20 percent of treated childhood spondylolisthesis is dysplastic.[viii]

Degenerative: When there is arthritis in the facet joints, they degenerate and lose their grip on the vertebra above or below and the vertebrae can slip forward. If you're an adult, this is the kind you're most likely to have. It is most commonly seen at the L4-L5 level, but can happen at other levels as well.

Traumatic: When you get thrown from a car or fall out of your tree house, you may break a bone in such a way that a vertebra can slip out of line.

Pathologic: This is caused by a tumor that weakens the bone and thus enables the slippage. This, as I say every time I mention tumors, is very rare.

Iatrogenic: Spondylolisthesis that occurs as an unfortunate result of a laminectomy.

We use a grading system to rate the severity of spondylolisthesis, with grade one being the least severe (grade zero being normal), and grade five being the most severe. The grade is determined by how far over the vertebra has slipped. If it has slipped less than 25 percent of the depth of the vertebra below, it's grade one. Grade two is 25–50 percent; grade three is 50–75 percent; grade four is 75–100 percent; and grade five is when the slipped vertebra has fallen completely off the vertebra below. We have a special name for grade five spondylolisthesis: spondyloptosis. It sounds very bad, and sometimes it is, but I've known patients to have it and not even know.

One of the misconceptions my patients often have about spondylolisthesis comes from that word "slip." They envision their vertebra constantly slipping back and forth over the one underneath. That's usually not what's going on. Most of the time, the vertebra moves out of line and stays there. It can, however, move farther out of line over time. There is only about a 5 percent chance of this, and it usually happens with children, whose skeletons are still growing.[ix] It's rare for spondylolisthesis to progress in an adult.

Degenerative spondylolisthesis in adults can also be seen in association with spinal stenosis. You can have one without the other, but they can also be seen together. The important thing to realize, if you have both, is that each causes different symptoms. Patients with both conditions may have both back pain (from the spondylolisthesis) and neurogenic claudication (from the stenosis).

Spondylolisthesis has a close relative in retrolisthesis, which is bone slippage in the other direction. Because the pressure on the lumbar spine pushes vertebrae forward, the usual slippage is for-

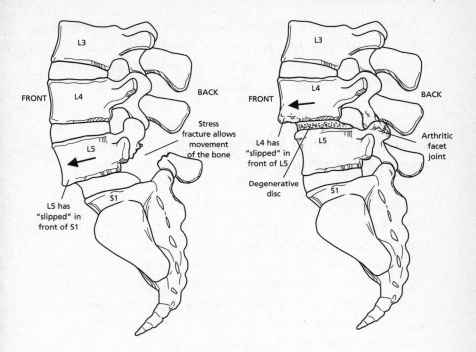

Two kinds of spondylolisthesis: Isthmic (left) is a stress fracture of
the pars interarticularis; degenerative (right) results from the
degeneration of the facet and disc.

ward, or anterolisthesis. Sometimes, though, a vertebra will slip
backward. It usually only slips a little bit, and almost never
causes trouble. It's important to know the difference between anterolisthesis (what we usually refer to as spondylolisthesis) and
retrolisthesis, because the treatments are very different: there's no
clear evidence that surgery is indicated for isolated retrolisthesis.

Symptoms and treatment options: They're the same for
spondylolysis and spondylolisthesis, with the obvious exception
that a direct pars repair doesn't apply.

Spondylolisthesis in children is beyond the scope of this book. For adults, when the pain is severe and unresponsive to the other treatments, surgery may be considered. There is abundant evidence that spinal fusion works for painful spondylolisthesis.

KYPHOSIS (FIXED SAGITTAL PLANE DEFORMITY, FLATBACK SYNDROME)

Kyphosis is when your lower back curves the wrong way. Normally, your lumbar spine curves into your body. If that curve (called lordosis) is removed, either by a disease or a surgical procedure, it has the effect of pushing your upper spine forward. The loss of the normal swayback is called kyphosis, and when it's bad enough to cause pain and functional limitations, you may need treatment.

Some kinds of scoliosis can be associated with kyphosis, as can a fracture of the vertebral body with angulation significant enough to change the curve of the spine. Some musculoskeletal conditions can cause it, as can an uncommon condition called ankylosing spondylitis (a kind of inflammatory arthritis that predominantly affects men).

Kyphosis can also be caused by surgery. It used to be that scoliosis surgery, which used implants called Harrington rods, was the most common cause; the procedure, necessary to correct the scoliosis, sometimes resulted in a severe kind of painful kyphosis in later life known as flatback syndrome. Surgeons now have better implants, and Harrington rods are a thing of the past. Spinal fusion, though, can occasionally cause kyphosis, in which case we call it fixed sagittal plane deformity (described in chapter 7).

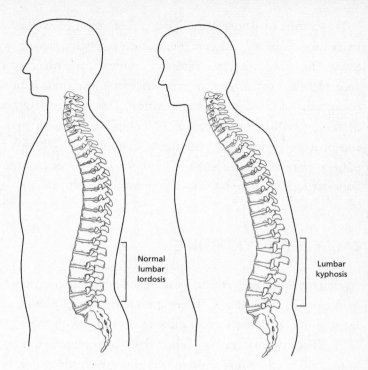

Kyphosis (right), or a bent-over spine, can result in severe pain and disability.

Symptoms: Back pain and fatigue are the primary symptoms. Because your spine isn't aligned correctly, just standing still is painful and tiring. I've seen patients who can't stand straight without bending their knees and flexing their hips to compensate for the absence of a normal swayback. Walking is also very difficult. If a patient comes to me with these symptoms and a history of spine surgery, I get a full-length standing X-ray of his spine to make the diagnosis. That's usually sufficient, although sometimes flexion and extension X-rays are also needed.

Treatment options: Although a combination of exercises, activity modification, and pain medication can help manage symptoms, the only way to restore alignment is with corrective surgery called osteotomy. In this procedure, the spine is broken, realigned and fused in a better position. This is an enormous undertaking with a large chance of complications and may not completely relieve your symptoms. Complications range from pain to paralysis, but, because kyphosis can be so painful and debilitating, for some patients the surgery is worth the risk.

FACET JOINT SYNDROME

Aside from the intervertebral disc, each vertebra connects to its neighbors in four places. There are two meeting points, called facet joints, with the vertebra above, and two with the vertebra below. Facet joints are also called the zygapophysial joints, or z joints. Like all joints, facet joints are susceptible to arthritis when cartilage wears down. They can also develop bone spurs and cysts.

Symptoms: Facet syndrome does not cause leg pain; you feel facet pain in your back, just as you feel pain in the knee from an arthritic knee. There's no easy way to differentiate facet joint pain from other back pain. The only way to determine whether it's your facet joint that's causing your pain is with a diagnostic injection (described in chapter 11).

Treatment options: Facet joint pain can often be managed with medication and exercise. If that doesn't work, a therapeutic injection of steroids into the joint may help you feel better. There is also a minimally invasive procedure called a neurotomy (see page 275), but its effectiveness is questionable.

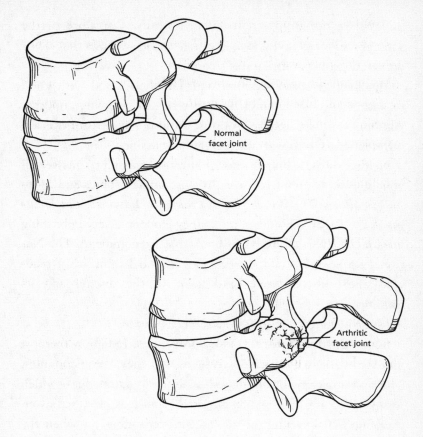

The facet joint (upper left) can become arthritic (lower right), with bone spurs, narrowing of the joint and loss of the articular cartilage.

SCOLIOSIS

Scoliosis is an abnormal lateral curvature of the spine. "Lateral" means the curve goes from side to side. Spines normally curve in at the lumbar level (lordosis) and out at the thoracic level (kyphosis), but they're not supposed to curve laterally. Curvature of the spine is measured in degrees, like angles, and scoliosis that is under ten degrees never requires treatment.

You may associate scoliosis with childhood, and with good reason. The most common kind develops in growing children. Although adults also have scoliosis, the issues and treatments are different enough to warrant separate discussions.

Neither of these discussions is thorough enough to answer all your questions about scoliosis. It's a complex topic, and *Stopping Scoliosis: The Whole Family Guide to Diagnosis and Treatment,* by Nancy Schommer and Nancy Hooper (Avery Publishing Group, 2002), is an excellent book that I recommend. The National Scoliosis Foundation endorses it, and I think it's a readable, thorough, accurate assessment of the disease and its treatments.

In the meantime, here are the scoliosis basics.

Scoliosis in children: Tumors, infections, radiation therapy, and some diseases can cause scoliosis, but they are uncommon. The vast majority of childhood scoliosis is idiopathic—which means we don't know what causes it—and it is classified as either infantile, juvenile, or adolescent, depending on when the child is diagnosed. The most common is the adolescent type.

In children, scoliosis is rarely painful. That is one reason scoliosis frequently isn't caught until the spine has developed a significant curve. If a child with scoliosis comes to me with back pain, it's a red flag, and I do a thorough investigation to find out if the scoliosis isn't idiopathic, and whether there's another condition along with it.

The most important reason we treat scoliosis in children is to prevent the curve from progressing, which it can do, especially while the skeleton is still growing. Once the skeleton stops

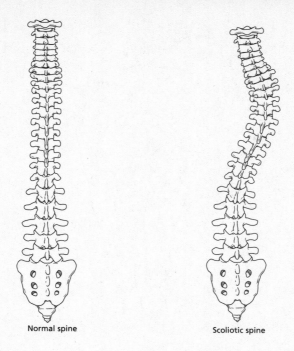

Normal spine   Scoliotic spine

The spine is normally straight when viewed from the back (left). In scoliosis (right), there is curvature to the side.

growing, the curve progresses much more slowly. Larger curves can cause pain later in life. One common misconception is that scoliosis compresses vital organs. This only happens with very large curves, of about ninety degrees or more.

Symptoms in children: There aren't any, which is why many school districts have screening programs. This method of detecting scoliosis, however, is controversial. The only way to tell for sure that a child has scoliosis is with an X-ray, but we can get a hint from doing a very simple test called the forward bending test. Stand behind the child, and have her bend over from the

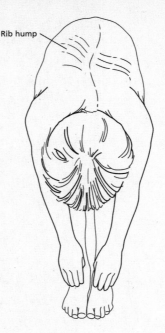

Rib hump

The forward bending test is the most common way doctors check for scoliosis in a physical exam. Notice the elevated ribs on one side and the depressed ribs on the other.

waist and touch her toes. If one shoulder or one side of the back looks higher than the other, it could be a sign of scoliosis. This test is by no means infallible. Some children with small curves will look uneven when they bend over, and some with big curves will look normal. Only an X-ray can identify scoliosis for sure.

Treatments for children: Since adolescent idiopathic scoliosis is by far the most common, I'm going to talk about its three treatment options: observation, bracing, and surgery.

I have a lot of patients who don't think of observation as a treatment, but it is. Observing doesn't mean ignoring. It means keeping track by seeing your doctor every three to six months and getting regular X-rays. Observation is what allows us to make intelligent choices about other kinds of treatment. In most cases, scoliosis is simply observed, and further intervention is not required.

The decision to brace is based on the size of the curve, its location, the speed with which it is changing, the age of the child, and the likelihood that the child will adjust to a brace. Doctors disagree about bracing. Some argue that the inconvenience and discomfort of a brace, coupled with the potential for stigma, outweigh the potential advantage. Which brings me to an important point: the best a brace can do is prevent a curve from getting bigger; curves can still progress despite bracing. Whether you brace or you don't, you still have to keep careful track of how the scoliosis is progressing, at least until the skeleton is fully grown, but you shouldn't even consider surgery for most types of idiopathic scoliosis in an adolescent until the curve is forty-five to fifty degrees. (There may be circumstances where surgery is appropriate in a younger child with a less pronounced curve.)

Surgical treatment for scoliosis is a spinal fusion with lots of screws, rods, and hooks. The issue of when to operate on adolescents for scoliosis is so difficult and complicated that I can't do it justice here. If you're facing that decision, read the book I referred to above.

Exercise doesn't qualify as a treatment, but it's important for scoliosis patients to stay active. I have met many parents who assumed that their kids couldn't exercise normally because of scoliosis, but that is not the case. Have your child go outside, run around, and be a kid! It won't make the scoliosis worse, and she will stay healthier.

CASE STUDY

COLLEEN first came to see me when she was about twelve, with scoliosis bad enough to warrant bracing. She wore the brace for two years, but that didn't stop her from playing the sports she loved—soccer and volleyball. After the two years, her curve made her a borderline candidate for surgery; together, we decided against it. Colleen and her parents were afraid that, after surgery, she couldn't be as active, and wouldn't be as good at volleyball, which she was playing very seriously. Because her condition was in the gray zone between needing surgery and not needing it, I agreed that she would be better off without it. She went on to play college volleyball, and even tried out for the Olympic team. Her scoliosis did not progress and she has never regretted her decision.

Scoliosis in adults: When we find scoliosis in an adult, it is possible because she had it in childhood and no one diagnosed it. Since we don't routinely X-ray every child's spine, we can't say for sure. Adults can also get a kind of scoliosis called degenerative scoliosis. Adult scoliosis progresses much more slowly than childhood scoliosis (less than one degree each year), and the primary indication for treatment is pain.

Symptoms in adults: Adult scoliosis can cause back pain. Adults who also have stenosis may also have leg pain.

Treatment options for adults: The decision of whether to treat scoliosis in adults is less straightforward than it is in adolescents, and has more to do with the degree of pain than the degree of the curve; the two often don't correlate. I've seen patients with fifty-degree curves in severe pain and patients with ninety-degree curves who are pain-free. And you know my mantra: if you can live with the pain, live without the surgery.

The factors in the decision to have surgery for scoliosis are different in children and adults. Scoliosis in children is painless, and the decision to operate is based on the size, location, and potential for further growth of the curve. In adults, those factors matter, but pain is also an important consideration.

SACROILIAC (SI) JOINT PROBLEMS

Your sacroiliac joint is called that because it's the connection between your sacrum and your ilium. That may not help you picture it, though, so let me give you a more graphic definition. The sacrum and ilium are two of the major bones in your pelvis, and the SI joint is where they meet just inside and up from the cheek of your buttock. There's one on each side, and they can cause low back pain.

If the SI joint is causing your problem, it's important to know it. While nonsurgical treatment for pain that originates in the lumbar spine is often the same regardless of which specific structure is causing it, treatment for pain that originates in the sacroiliac joint is often site-specific.

The SI joint can break, get infected, or the bones around it can be invaded by cancer—the same emergencies that can affect the rest of the spine. In those cases, the SI joint is treated in the same way as the spine.

Sometimes, though, when the SI joint hurts, the problem is one of the inflammatory kinds of arthritis, like ankylosing spondylitis. For reasons that aren't completely clear, certain types of inflammatory arthritis tend to involve the SI joint. (There are also degenerative kinds of arthritis, like osteoarthritis, that don't have a particular predilection for the SI joint.)

Human anatomy makes it difficult to see the SI joint clearly with an X-ray. Many problems won't show up. You'll probably need a CT scan, MRI scan, bone scan, or all three. I can also tell, with a fair degree of certainty, whether your pain comes from the SI joint by doing a diagnostic injection. If I numb the joint and the pain goes away, it's a good bet that it's the source of the pain.

Symptoms: The symptom of SI joint problems is pain in the buttock, and it's difficult to distinguish it from referred pain that you feel in the buttock but that originates in the back. If you and your doctor suspect SI joint involvement, a diagnostic injection may be in order.

Treatment options: With the exception of emergencies, the treatment of SI joint pain is primarily nonsurgical. There are the usual pain-fighting strategies, such as exercise, physical therapy, and medication, and there are injections. Because we can't always identify exactly what's causing SI joint pain, we sometimes inject steroidal anti-inflammatory medications, hoping they will help. Fusion is not recommended unless the pain is severe and unresponsive to other treatment options.

DISCOGENIC LOW BACK PAIN

Discogenic pain is simply pain that is thought to originate in a disc, and there are various diagnoses that are used to explain it. They include (but aren't limited to):

degenerative disc disease
black disc
internal disc disruption (IDD)

These diagnoses have several things in common, but the most important factor they share is uncertainty. If you're diagnosed with discogenic pain, you need to know that there's no consensus in the spine community that there is such a thing. When we say pain is discogenic, it's a guess. We don't know for sure how discs (unless they're herniated and pressing on a nerve) cause pain, or whether a particular disc is the culprit.

Another element all these diagnoses have in common is that they rest on "abnormalities" found on tests. But remember that if we look at test results from people with no back pain, we often find many of the same abnormalities.

The one and only symptom of all of the discogenic diagnoses is low back pain, and the treatment options are also the same. Try everything—exercise, activity modification, medication, physical therapy, acupuncture—until you find what works.

Although the treatment may be the same, it's important to understand the specifics of what you've been diagnosed with. The first two diagnoses—degenerative disc disease and black disc—are a little different from internal disc disruption and internal derangement of the disc (which are synonyms, and both abbreviated IDD), so I want to divide this category into two subcategories.

DEGENERATIVE DISC DISEASE AND BLACK DISC

To understand what a degenerated disc is, let's go back to the jelly donut analogy. If you let the donut sit out too long, the jelly will dry out and harden, and the donut will shrink. That's what happens with a degenerated disc. It loses its water content, dries out, and shrinks. The proteins and cartilage of the disc change as that happens, and your disc loses its elasticity and ability to absorb shock.

A degenerated disc shows up on an X-ray in several ways. Although the X-ray doesn't see the disc itself, it sees the space that the disc takes up. If that space is much smaller than it's supposed to be, it means the disc has shrunk. Additionally, because the disc is no longer cushioning the vertebrae around it, the bones above and below the disc start to move abnormally. This can cause bone spurs and a condition called sclerosis, in which white, hard bone is formed at the end plate, where the vertebral body connects to the disc. Both of these are visible on an X-ray.

There can be more subtle findings too. You might, for example, have a black disc, which appears on an MRI scan. When discs begin to degenerate, they lose water, and, since water shows up as white on an MRI, a normal, hydrated disc looks white. Once the disc starts to lose moisture, the intensity of the white decreases, and when much of the water is gone, it shows up as black.

A black disc sounds very ominous, but it's really not scary at all. If you're over forty, chances are that a test will find either a

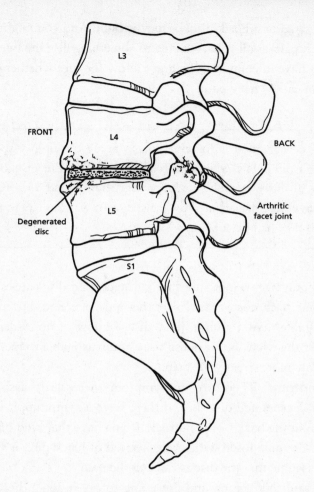

FRONT

BACK

L3

L4

L5

S1

Degenerated disc

Arthritic facet joint

Side view of the lumbar spine shows an L4-L5 degenerated lumbar disc. Note the loss of height of the disc compared to the healthier discs above and below. Also shown is an associated degenerated facet joint of L4-L5.

degenerated or a black disc, or maybe both. And you might have no back pain at all. That's a clue to something else the two conditions have in common. We don't know for sure whether either of them causes back pain.

> **Disc degeneration is for everyone.** A study of autopsy specimens from published reports found that 36 percent of lumbar discs in thirty-year-olds had disc degeneration and 93 percent of discs were degenerated by age sixty.[x] (It was too late to find out if they had back pain.)

Not only are we not sure that a degenerated disc causes pain, but some back doctors speculate that a degenerated disc may be more stable than a plump, juicy disc. I know of no evidence to support this view, but it doesn't seem unreasonable to me. Until we know more, treat your pain.

Symptoms: There are no symptoms necessarily associated with a degenerated disc. But, if there were a symptom, it would be pain in the back or the buttock. If you have that kind of pain, and you're diagnosed with a degenerated or black disc, it's natural to assume that the disc is causing the pain.

I've said this before, and I'm going to say it again, because I think it is important for you to understand: It is very difficult to pinpoint the source of pain, and it's way too easy to take an X-ray or do an MRI scan, find an anomaly, and attribute the pain to the anomaly. Do not fall into this trap.

Treatment options: If you have low back pain and a diagnosis of degenerative disc disease, you should be thinking about treating the pain, not treating the disease. The most commonly used surgical treatments for degenerative disc disease are fusion (and, recently, artificial disc replacement) and intradiscal electrothermal therapy (IDET), in which heat is applied directly to the disc in the hope of killing the nerves that transmit the pain. (Read all about it on page 270.)

Surgery, however, does not seem to work any better than simply leaving well enough alone. According to an overview of the treatment of degenerative disc disease published in the medical journal *Spine* in 2003, "It is not established in the literature that any of these procedures, including fusion techniques, are superior to natural history or non-operative treatment."[xi] There you have it.

INTERNAL DISC DISRUPTION (IDD)

IDD is a very controversial diagnosis, identified by findings on MRI scans and confirmed with discograms (see page 85). The diagnostic process begins with the MRI, which your doctor will use to check the annulus (the firm outer part of the disc) for tears, fissures, and what are called high-intensity zones. This is also where the controversy begins. Some doctors don't believe these findings can be linked to pain. Others do. I am firmly in the first camp. Those same doctors also call IDD by another name— internal derangement of the disc. I tell my patients that IDD also stands for Impossible to Diagnose this Disease.

People who believe in the link to pain do so because the outer part of the annulus contains nerves (although the inner part doesn't), and a tear has the potential to irritate the nerve either mechanically or by allowing a leakage of chemicals. This is merely speculation. As with herniation, many people with no back pain—as many as 24 percent—have high-intensity zones and annular tears or fissures.[xii]

If your doctor believes in IDD, he'll confirm the "abnormalities" he found on the MRI with a painful, invasive test called a discogram. The theory behind the test is that if you pump fluid into a disc that is suspected of being the source of pain, it will reproduce your pain. If the test is painful, therefore, the conclusion is that the disc is the source of your problem. That conclusion, though, is suspect. Because a discogram is the only test we have that's supposed to tell us if pain is discogenic, there is absolutely no way to confirm the results. In fact, an award-winning study found that people who have those "abnormalities" and no back pain are just as likely to have positive discogram results as people who have those abnormalities and do have back pain. The researchers concluded that the idea that high intensity zones are indicators of symptomatic IDD is "seriously flawed."[xiii]

Yet doctors rely on discograms to diagnose IDD. In doing so, they're piling controversy on top of controversy. They're using a questionable test to support a questionable diagnosis. Nevertheless, IDD diagnoses are on the rise. Not a week goes by that I don't see a patient seeking a second opinion for an IDD diagnosis.

> **Discogenic pain** is low back pain postulated to come from an intervertebral disc. Because it is difficult to prove that anyone's pain is coming from a particular disc, surgery to cure the pain is unpredictable.

I believe that IDD is a by-product of the frustration doctors have in treating a problem whose only symptom is pain. It is this frustration—seeing a patient who clearly needs help, but whose tests show ambiguous findings—that can lay the groundwork for treatment that doesn't work.

Symptoms: The kind of pain for which IDD is usually invoked is chronic low back pain, sometimes with buttock pain, that is aggravated by activity. That may sound definitive, but think about it. If you've tried physical therapy, and it didn't work, your doctor can say, "Aha! It must be IDD because your pain didn't respond to physical therapy." IDD isn't a predictive diagnosis. Your doctor doesn't look at the MRI results and say, "You have IDD and you can expect to have pain that doesn't respond to physical therapy." Instead, IDD is a diagnosis designed to fit the symptoms of a patient with difficult, persistent, unresponsive back pain. It is a diagnosis of exclusion.

Treatment options: Doctors who believe that IDD causes pain also believe that fusion surgery can fix it. Because I don't believe that these MRI findings can be linked to pain, I don't believe that surgery should be the treatment. My advice is to treat the pain, not the finding on your MRI.

ACUTE LOW BACK PAIN

Back pain that gets better in six weeks or less is defined as acute. If you've been told that this is what you have, you should know that it's code for "We have no idea." It could be caused by a strain of a muscle or a sprain in a ligament—neither of which have precise definitions. It could also be a flare-up of underlying degenerative arthritis. Some doctors refer to acute low back pain as "idiopathic," which just means we don't know the cause. By any name, acute low back pain is so common that it's the second most common reason people seek medical advice (after the common cold). Unfortunately, or fortunately, depending on how you look at it, the only way you know you have it is that it gets better.

I don't want you to despair if you've been told that this is what you have. You may be better off than your neighbor, your coworker, or your nephew who's gotten a more specific diagnosis. Once you understand that there's no way to pinpoint the cause of your pain, you're much less likely to end up getting treatment that doesn't work. That's particularly important if the treatment in question is surgery.

The next four chapters are about the many nonsurgical treatments that my patients—and clinical studies—have found to be effective. Chances are very good that you'll find options that work for you.

ENDNOTES

i D. F. Fardon, MD, and P. C. Milette, MD. "Nomenclature and Classification of Lumbar Disc Pathology: Recommendations of the Combined Task Forces of the North American Spine Society, American Society of Spine Radiology, and American Society of Neuroradiology." *Spine* 26, no. 5 (2001), pp. E93–E113.

ii M. C. Jensen, M. N. Brant-Zawadzki, N. Obuchowski, et al., "Magnetic Resonance Imaging of the Lumbar Spine in People Without Back Pain," *New England Journal of Medicine* 331, no. 2 (1994), pp. 69–73.

iii Fardon and Milette, "Nomenclature and Classification."

iv S. D. Boden, D. O. Davis, T. S. Dina, et al., "Abnormal Magnetic-Resonance Scans of the Lumbar Spine in Asymptomatic Subjects: A Prospective Investigation," *Journal of Bone and Joint Surgery (Am.)* 72, no. 3 (1990), pp. 403–08.

v Fardon and Milette, "Nomenclature and Classification."

vi J. A. Saal, J. S. Saal, R. J. Herzog, "The Natural History of Lumbar Intervertebral Disc Extrusions Treated Nonoperatively," *Spine* 15, no. 7 (1990), pp. 683–86.

vii J. E. Lonstein, "Spondylolisthesis in Children: Cause, Natural History, and Management," *Spine* 24, no. 24 (1999), pp. 2640–48.

viii Ibid.

ix Ibid.

x J. A. Miller, C. Schmatz, A. B. Schultz, "Lumbar Disc Degeneration: Correlation with Age, Sex, and Spine Level in 600 Autopsy Specimens," *Spine* 13, no. 12 (1988), pp. 173–78.

xi H. An, et al., "Summary Statement: Emerging Techniques."

xii E. Carragee, J. Paragioudakis, S. Khurana, et al., "2000 Volvo Award Winner in Clinical Studies: Lumbar High-Intensity Zone and Discography in Subjects Without Low Back Problems," *Spine* 25, no. 23 (2000), pp. 2987–92.

xiii Ibid.

DODGING THE KNIFE

Alternatives to Surgery

Chapter 8

EXERCISE

When you weigh surgical treatment options for back pain, the specter of complications looms large. There are infections, hematomas, and blood clots. There's paralysis and pain and instability. There's even death. When you consider exercise, though, the equation is a little different. There is certainly the possibility that it won't help you, but the side effects are fitness, strength, and weight loss.

And those are just the physical side effects; there are mental ones too. Exercise helps fight stress and depression, neither of which is good for back pain. I've also found that exercise helps to give my patients a sense of control over their pain. They no longer feel like they're enslaved by it. Taking control by exercising your pain into submission can be positively exhilarating.

In short, you can't go wrong with exercise. While it's possible that pain can be exacerbated by exercise, it's so much more likely that it will be alleviated that it's foolish not to try it. I've found that patients who are resistant to exercise often have attitudes that are holdovers from the days when bed rest was thought to be the best cure for back pain. Back in those olden days, we had the idea that the spine was delicate, and if something went wrong it was to be pampered. Although those days are long gone, there's still vestigial fear lingering in some patients. If it hurts to move, they just can't believe that moving is a good idea. Well, it is.

Let me prove to you the power of fear and pain. It involves a very simple and particularly compelling study done in Norway, and published in 1995. Because Norway has a system of national health insurance, the government can track everyone who takes more than eight weeks of sick leave from work. After the eighth week, Norwegians need a special certificate, and the researchers collected about eight hundred subjects who got such a certificate for low back pain. They randomly assigned those eight hundred either to a control group, which got conventional nonsurgical treatment (which could have been anything; the study doesn't specify), and an intervention group, which got two medical appointments, one for testing and one for consultation. Regardless of the test results, all the subjects in the intervention group got the same consultation. Here's a description of what they were told, and I think it gets across the spirit of the study:

> The patients were told how a possible crack in a disc can cause an inflammation . . . and lead to stiffness and pain. . . . They were also given the assurance that light activity would not further injure the disc or any other structure . . . and that it was more likely that it rather would enhance the repair process. . . . The point that the worst thing they could do to their backs was to be to [sic] careful, was strongly emphasized. . . . [They] were told to mobilize the lumbar spine by light activity. . . . Great emphasis was put on the effort to remove fear about LBP and focus on sickness behavior.[i]

Basically, they were told that back pain was nothing to be afraid of, that it often went away all by itself, and that activity was the best thing for it. That's all. Yet, two hundred days later,

70 percent of that intervention group was back at work, compared with only 40 percent of the control group. I'm sure the encouragement to exercise made a difference to the intervention group; exercise has been shown to be effective for back pain. But I'm going to go out on a limb here and speculate that the biggest factor in the recovery of the subjects in the intervention group was their attitude. They were led to believe that back pain was something they could recover from, that they shouldn't worry too much, and that they should move around. Sure enough, most of them recovered to the point where they could go back to work.

Don't let the fact that I find this study interesting and useful make you believe that I think low back pain is something trivial that doesn't require care. Quite the contrary; I think it is critical that doctors take it seriously and work closely with their patients from the very first office visit. Part of that work, though, is setting expectations and making lifestyle changes. If the expectations are of recovery, and the lifestyle changes are conducive to it, your chances of success are maximized.

So maybe it isn't fear that is holding you back; maybe something else is. Some patients are simply hiding behind that slim chance that moving and stretching and strengthening will make them worse rather than better. Their real objection is the objection that we all have to exercise—it's hard. It takes time and effort. You have to do it regularly, and it's not always pleasant. You should step up to it, though. Exercise is one of the best treatments we have, both because it's one of the most effective and because its side effects are beneficial rather than harmful.

Once you decide to try exercise, the question is which exercise? The answer is that it almost doesn't matter. There have been numerous studies investigating everything from yoga to weight lifting, and almost all of them show some benefit for chronic back pain. An analysis of sixty-one of those studies was published in the *Annals of Internal Medicine* in 2005, and the authors concluded: "These trials provide strong evidence that exercise therapy is at least as effective as other conservative interventions and conflicting evidence that exercise therapy is more effective than other treatments for chronic low back pain."[ii] In other words, it's definitely as good as other treatments, and it might be better. There you have it. Sign up today.

Note that the authors specified *chronic* low back pain. Acute pain is a different story. If your pain comes on very suddenly, it's less likely that exercise will help. On the other hand, it probably won't hurt, and I urge you to try it anyway. The research I cite in this chapter, though, is for chronic low back pain.

MAKING SENSE OF THE OPTIONS

Although it doesn't matter much what kind of exercise program you choose, I want you to understand the basics of the choices. There are four components of exercise, and different programs mix and match them. The parts are: range of motion, stretching, strengthening, and aerobic conditioning. Range of motion exercises are for the joint. They're supposed to increase the range of motion. Stretching is for muscles, tendons, and ligaments. Strengthening is for muscles. Aerobic conditioning is for cardiovascular fitness.

Most exercise programs that target back pain are heavy on the strengthening and aerobic components. If the muscles around your spine and in your abdomen are strong, they help the spine do its job. The rationale for aerobic conditioning is a little more holistic. If it's good for the heart and lungs, it's good for the back. While we can't say for sure that adding the other two components—stretching and range of motion—to the program increases its effectiveness, the golden rule of exercise still applies: it might help your back, and it's good for you anyway.

Remember that golden rule as you make your choices. Our understanding of how and why exercise fights back pain isn't nearly good enough to say that strengthening this muscle is better than strengthening that muscle, or that yoga is better than Pilates, or that swimming is better than Rollerblading. If you're trying to find out which exercise program is the best, you're out of luck. Besides, "best" would just mean that it was more effective for more people than other programs. That would be no guarantee that it would be best for you.

I want you to take the news that there's no "best" as good news. If there were a "best," and you found that you hated doing it, you'd be in a bad spot. But bestlessness means you have choices, and you can find the kind of exercise regimen that you like, that you can stick with, and that makes you feel better. Here are some of the kinds of exercise that I've known patients to benefit from:

walking
running
swimming
Rollerblading
elliptical trainer use
yoga
Pilates
water aerobics
bicycling
circuit training

Any of those can be supplemented by back-specific exercises. There are a lot of those out there, and no good way to choose among them. One book that outlines a back program I like is *Back RX: A Fifteen-Minute-a-Day Yoga- and Pilates-Based Program to End Low Back Pain*, by Vijay Vad, M.D., and Hilary Hinzmann (Gotham Books, 2004). On the Web, there's a good overview of exercise at www.aaos.org.

All of these are things you can do on your own, no doctor required. When you get a doctor involved, exercise has another name—physical therapy.

PHYSICAL THERAPY

If you've ever wondered how physical therapy is different from good old-fashioned exercise, you're in good company. A lot of my patients ask the question, and the answer is that physical therapy *is* exercise. It's a directed program, designed specifically to increase function and decrease pain through exercise.

There are almost as many kinds of physical therapies as there are physical therapists, and there's not a lot to go on if you're trying to choose among them. As with other kinds of exercise, though, it probably doesn't matter much which kind you choose (with a couple of exceptions, which I'll get to). It seems that any program of regular, directed physical therapy can help reduce back pain and increase function. Some of the most common programs are:

- hip-, hamstring-, and calf-stretching programs;
- Williams' flexion exercises, which emphasize strengthening the abdominal muscles;
- McKenzie extension exercises, which work on the back muscles;

- core stabilization/strengthening programs, which teach abdominal and paraspinal muscle strengthening; and
- dynamic stabilization training, which adds movement to the above program.

All of these require a prescription from a doctor. It can be any kind of doctor—it doesn't have to be a spine surgeon or even a physiatrist; your internist can prescribe it. The kind of physical therapy you choose may have a lot to do with your doctor's preferences, and those preferences may be based more on his knowledge of local providers than on any clinical research comparing one method to another. And that's just fine, since there isn't much of that research, and what there is isn't definitive.

I have one criterion for physical therapy: it has to be exercise. But wait, you say, didn't I just explain that physical therapy *is* exercise? Yes, I did. And it is, most of the time. Increasingly, though, some new kinds of treatment that *aren't* exercise are being introduced into physical therapy regimens.

Modalities: That's the catchall name for the no-exercise parts of physical therapy that run the gamut from ultrasound to massage, and include transcutaneous electrical nerve stimulation (TENS), hot and cold packs, deep tissue release, and spinal traction.

Modalities are fun, they feel good, they don't require effort . . . and they do nothing. Or close to nothing, at any rate—there's no evidence that any of them relieve pain or increase function, the two goals of physical therapy. Their use in physical therapy is probably driven both by the fact that patients enjoy them and that physical therapists can fit in more patients doing modalities than doing exercise because modalities don't require as much one-on-one time.

There's also no evidence that modalities do any harm, of course, so you may be wondering why I take issue with them. While it's true that they don't cause harm in themselves, the danger is in what patients *aren't* doing while they're using modalities. They're not exercising, and it's exercise that makes physical therapy effective. If you like modalities, there's no harm in spending five minutes on them at the beginning or end of your session, but the bulk of your time with the PT should be spent exercising. If your therapist insists on them exclusively, get a new therapist.

Don't let the fact that this chapter is short lead you to believe that exercise is unimportant. I could have made this chapter even shorter (Exercise: Get Some!), and it still would have been one of the most important in the book. As a surgeon who wants back pain patients to avoid surgery, I rank exercise as one of my best pain management tools. If you're a back pain patient who wants to avoid surgery, the best thing you can do for your back is to get moving.

ENDNOTES

i A. Indahl, L. Velund, O. Reikeraas, "Good Prognosis for Low Back Pain When Left Untampered: A Randomized Clinical Trial," *Spine* 20, no. 4 (1995), pp. 473–77.

ii J. A. Hayden, et al., "Meta-Analysis: Exercise Therapy for Nonspecific Low Back Pain," *Annals of Internal Medicine* 142 (2005), pp. 765–75.

Chapter 9

ALTERNATIVE TREATMENTS

S o, if surgery isn't the answer, what is? That's probably the single most important question my patients ask me, and the answer is that it could be almost anything from acupuncture to a good night's sleep. Although I am a surgeon, I much prefer to help my patients manage their conditions by other means, each of which could merit its own book. In fact, they have merited their own books—and Web sites, magazine articles, and television shows. If I covered each of the alternatives exhaustively, this book would be impractically long, heavy, and expensive, so I've chosen instead to touch on each one briefly and to point you to other sources of information for more details.

If you've read the previous chapter on exercise, you already know what I believe is the most important nonsurgical treatment we have. Exercise is almost always my first recommendation. Although I call the treatments in this chapter alternative, I want to emphasize that they're not alternatives to exercise. All of these (with the exception of bed rest, but more on that later) can be tried in conjunction with exercise, which is the way I urge you to try them unless you've been specifically prohibited from exercising. Many of you will be tempted not to. Exercise is hard and many of these alternatives are easier.

> **Exercise is the first line of defense.** "Alternative" treatments are alternatives to surgery, not to exercise. Try them in addition to an exercise program.

But I think exercise is the most constructive alternative to surgery there is, because it is effective and because it's just plain good for you. That said, some of these other choices work well for many patients, and are worth trying.

There is very little strong clinical evidence for the efficacy of most of these. The best I can say is that they all seem to work at least a little. There are many studies with many flaws, and the outcomes are often equivocal. The researchers find no difference among treatments, or small differences that don't mean much in light of the methodological problems with the studies. The popularity of these treatments has been built primarily on anecdotal evidence, which is abundant. It may be that, in a prospective, randomized, controlled, double-blind clinical trial (the best type of scientific study we can do), none of them would pan out. But I don't evaluate most of these techniques with the same rigor that I evaluate the effectiveness of surgical procedures for one simple reason: there's not much downside. And back pain is so tied up with a patient's state of mind, his temperament, his beliefs, and his expectations that I encourage you to try any harmless treatment you have even a mild curiosity about.

The key word there is "harmless." There are "alternative" treatments that may not be harmless. If there is a potential for harm, even if it's small, you have to take a closer look than you would at treatments that are completely safe. There are herbs used for back pain that can have serious side effects, so if they don't work for back pain there's no reason to take them. If stress management doesn't work for back pain, though, the worst-case scenario is better stress management with the same back pain as before.

Because that's an important distinction, I've divided this chapter into three sections: No Risk, Small Risk, and Significant Risk. Feel free to try any of the No Risk treatments because there is—I know you get it by now—no risk. Exercise a little more caution with the Small Risk treatments. If they weren't essentially safe I wouldn't include them in this chapter, but I would be remiss if I didn't tell you about the downside. I reserved the Significant Risk category for treatments that I regard as doing more harm than good in many circumstances.

No Risk	Small Risk	Significant Risk
Modification of activity	Acupuncture	Braces, corsets, and lumbar supports
Stress management	Herbal medications	Bed rest
Better sleep	Chiropractic and osteo-pathic manipulation	
Weight loss		
Smoking cessation		

NO RISK

MODIFICATION OF ACTIVITY

There's an old joke where a patient goes to see the doctor. He raises his arm way above his ahead and winces in pain. "Doc," he says, "it hurts when I do this with my arm." "Then don't do that," replies the doctor. Dumb joke, good lesson. If it hurts when you do a specific activity, stop doing that activity—or at least cut back. If it hurts to sit for more than an hour, you don't need a doctor to tell you to get up every forty-five minutes or so.

There are times when that's impossible. If it hurts when you lift, and you're a baggage handler, this is a solution that's not going to work for you. There are also times when you just don't want to do this. I've learned the hard way not to tell golfers they can't golf. The best I can do is gently suggest that nine holes twice a week might work better than eighteen holes once.

CASE STUDY

BETSY is a runner who strained her back. She could run, but it hurt. She was distressed because she had eight weeks to go before her first marathon. She'd been training for months, and was very worried about losing her hard-won cardiovascular conditioning. I gave her a prescription—for swimming and Rollerblading. Two weeks later, she was back on her feet. Six weeks after that, she successfully completed her marathon.

Note that this is *modification* of activity, not *cessation* of activity. It's very important to keep moving, so make sure you substitute an activity you can do comfortably for the one that's uncomfortable.

This may sound like it's too simple a strategy to work for serious pain, but I've seen it work time after time. Modifying your activity doesn't cure the pain, it just gives it a chance to go away by itself—which most back pain eventually does.

STRESS MANAGEMENT

Back pain isn't just about your back. It's also about your head. Stress and pain management don't mix well. I'm often asked whether stress can cause back problems, and the answer is that we don't know. We do know, though, that stress can make any kind of pain worse.

There's a very-well-known doctor who writes about the connection between the mind and the body and how stress and tension play a role in back pain. He's John Sarno, and many back pain sufferers swear by his books, two of which are *The Mindbody Prescription* (Warner Books, 1998), and *Mind Over Back Pain* (Berkley Books, 1999). I recommend either of them.

BETTER SLEEP

A bad night's sleep can make for a rough day under the best of circumstances. When your back hurts, it's worse; sleep deprivation exacerbates pain. Getting more, better sleep is hard. When I have insomniac patients, I try to find ways to get them to sleep better by changing habits, reducing stress, and exercising. As a last resort, I sometimes consider medication, but that is a short-term solution that doesn't tackle the root of the problem. There are, however, new sleep drugs that work very well, and if you're sleeping badly, you may want to talk to your doctor about them if other strategies aren't working.

WEIGHT LOSS

There's no definitive proof that weight contributes to back pain, but I don't let that stop me from recommending that my overweight patients slim down. Intuitively, it makes sense that extra weight is bad for your back. The heavier you are, the harder your spine has to work to keep you upright, bend you over, or get you up from a chair. But even if extra weight doesn't exacerbate back problems, there are too many good reasons to lose it for any doctor to miss an opportunity to help a patient work on diet and exercise.

I have seen patients' back pain improve with weight loss, but I'm certainly ready to acknowledge that the change may be more psychological than physical. Losing weight changes the way people think about themselves. Their attitudes about everything from their personal relationships to their careers change, and for the better. With a brighter outlook, almost everything improves, including back pain.

There are shelves and shelves of weight-loss books at the library and the bookstore, and it's hard to figure out which might be helpful. I do have one gauge that turns out to be pretty accurate. The farther the book gets away from the basics of weight loss—eat less, exercise more—the less likely it is to do you any good.

My personal favorite diet books are the *Volumetrics* series, by Barbara Rolls. Their premise is that if you eat foods that are low in calories but high-volume, you'll stay fuller longer on less food. Rolls emphasizes foods like vegetables, soups, and popcorn, and steers you clear of calorie-dense foods that are high in sugar and fat. It's a sensible, effective plan.

SMOKING CESSATION

As with weight loss, there are a million reasons to stop smoking. Let me give you one more: there's hard evidence that says it'll help your back. Smoking can cause premature degeneration of the intervertebral discs. Smokers have a higher incidence of low back pain, herniated discs, and osteoporosis.

If that weren't enough, there are also smoking-specific problems with any surgical procedure because the risks inherent in anesthesia and incisions are increased in smokers. It's even more important to stop smoking if you're considering a spinal fusion, since smoking inhibits bone formation.

You've heard it from your family, your friends, your doctors, and, in all probability, strangers on the street. Now you're hearing it from me. Stop smoking.

SMALL RISK

ACUPUNCTURE

Acupuncture has the distinction of being the oldest treatment on this list, dating back to perhaps 1500 B.C. Three and a half millennia later, though, its effectiveness is still being debated, in the spine field and elsewhere.

There have been many studies of acupuncture for back pain, and both their quality and results are all over the map. A 1999 overview of the research concluded that acupuncture wasn't effective for back pain,[i] but a 2005 review, which included several large, well-administered studies that had been done since the earlier review, concluded that acupuncture did work, at least in the short run, for low back pain. It doesn't seem to work any better than other therapies, but the authors found enough evidence to say definitively that it works better than no treatment or than sham treatments.[ii]

Why it works is another question. There's not much scientific support for the traditional Chinese explanation, and many doctors and scientists attribute acupuncture's ability to relieve pain solely to the placebo effect. For purposes of this discussion, it doesn't matter much. I know many patients who swear by acupuncture, and others who have found it doesn't work at all.

There is some risk involved, primarily of infections and nerve damage, but it's small. If you're interested in acupuncture, don't let those risks deter you.

HERBAL MEDICATIONS

Many of my patients have reported improvements they attribute to herbal supplements. There is very little in the way of well-conducted research on the effectiveness of most herbs, but some of them may work—at least a little. Many, many herbs are alleged to have pain-fighting properties, and most are low-risk, so it can't hurt to try them.

An excellent source for more information on herbal supplements is www.nlm.nih.gov/medlineplus/druginformation.html. Not only does this site tell you all about the herbs—properties, side effects, contraindications—it lists each condition the herb is supposed to be good for and rates the quality of the research supporting that contention.

Although they are mostly safe, herbs do have active ingredients, and there is the potential both for unpleasant (and occasionally dangerous) side effects and interaction with other medication. Make sure you tell your doctor if you're taking any supplement at all, herbs included.

CHIROPRACTIC AND OSTEOPATHIC MANIPULATION

Chiropractic treatments are, after exercise, the most popular pain relief avenue my patients choose. And they're not alone. At least 10 percent of Americans visit the chiropractor every year, primarily for back and neck problems.[iii] Despite the lack of evidence for the effectiveness of chiropractic treatments over the long term, chiropractors can help low back pain in the short run.

There are other treatments that involve physical manipulation of the spine but aren't, strictly speaking, chiropractic. One is osteopathic manipulation. It's done by doctors of osteopathy, who have rigorous, extensive educational backgrounds comparable to those of medical doctors. The manipulation is slightly different in its goal. Theories vary, but osteopathic manipulation is supposed to optimize blood circulation, and chiropractic manipulation is supposed to improve nerve transmission. Whether either accomplishes these goals is anybody's guess, but they can both help with back pain to about an equal extent.

That extent is small. There's a lot of research, but most of it is poorly done, and the results vary. My best synopsis of all the research is this: For both acute and chronic low back pain, short-term physical manipulation of the spine is better than sham therapy but has no clinically significant advantages over seeing your family physician, analgesics, physical therapy, exercises, or back school.[iv]

If you're wondering why chiropractic sessions work, I'm afraid I can't help you. I don't know either. Chiropractors manipulate the spine, and claim to align everything so that pain is minimized, but studies of X-rays taken before and after chiropractic sessions show no change in alignment of the sacroiliac joint.[v] It's possible that chiropractic and other manipulative therapies work because you get to talk about your problems with someone who listens to you. It's a hands-on therapy that most people find pleasant and relaxing, and it's a general feel-good experience.

Don't confuse chiropractic treatments with physical therapy. When you see the chiropractor, you have things done to you. When you see the physical therapist, you do things. Going to the chiropractor is easier and, for many people, more enjoyable than going to the physical therapist, but don't substitute the first for the second. Physical therapy is proven to help manage long-term back pain. Chiropractic treatments are not. Taken together, though, they may be just the combination that works. It does for many of my patients. To facilitate the combination, some chiropractic offices also offer physical therapy, and vice versa. That's both a convenience and a reminder to do both.

Many of my patients swear by their chiropractor, and I encourage them to continue their treatments as long as they're helpful. Once your pain stops, though, there's no reason to continue to go. Although some chiropractors promote "maintenance pro-grams," which allegedly keep your pain from coming back, there's no evidence they accomplish that goal.

You should know that there isn't evidence that chiropractic treatment helps in the long run, but if you can afford it, and you find it useful, the only reason to stop seeing your chiropractor is if your pain goes away.

I will add a caveat about modalities, the treatments like heat therapy, ultrasound, and electrical muscle stimulation that are common adjuncts both to physical therapy and chiropractic treat-ments. The evidence is that they don't work, and it doesn't make sense to pay good money to undergo them. A 2002 study com-pared chiropractic treatment with and without these modalities, and found very little difference. The study had a fundamental flaw because if the modalities group believed that their treatments would help, they might indeed see more improvement than the chiropractic-only group. And the modalities group did see slightly more pain relief in the two-to-six-week range, but it disappeared at six months. The authors concluded: "Physical modalities used by chiropractors in this managed-care organization did not appear to be effective in the treatment of patients with LBP, although a small short-term benefit for some patients cannot be ruled out."[vi]

There is, however, a reason that chiropractors are in the Small Risk section of this chapter. Most chiropractic risk comes from manipulation of the neck, rather than the lumbar spine. None-theless, many chiropractors treat the whole back for low back pain, so I would be remiss if I didn't mention the risk. Neck manipulation has been known to cause artery damage, nerve in-jury, fracture, and even stroke. Those risks are small; they're in the realm of one in one million sessions,[vii] and I think the potential benefits outweigh them for many patients. The exceptions are patients with osteoporosis or a history of vertebral fractures, vascular disease, nerve injury, or any other condition that might be affected by manipulation of the spine. For them, chiropractic manipulation could cause injury.

If you're thinking about seeing a chiropractor and you don't have one of the conditions I just mentioned, give it a try. If you find that the pain doesn't respond to treatment or gets worse, stop. Ditto if you start having symptoms like weakness or paralysis, fevers or chills, weight loss, or a change in bowel or bladder habits. It isn't that chiropractic treatments cause those things; it's that those things might be a sign that something serious is wrong. Chiropractors can't fix serious problems, and you need to see a doctor.

SIGNIFICANT RISK

BRACES, CORSETS, AND LUMBAR SUPPORTS

What's risky about a brace? You'd be surprised.

In medspeak, a brace is called an orthosis, and it comes in many different varieties, from a hard plastic shell to elastic supports. Some are prescription and others are available in any medical supply store. The problem with many of them is that, for many conditions, their effectiveness hasn't been established. They may help spinal fusions heal (I talk about that more specifically in chapter 13: Spinal Fusion), and they do help slow the progression of scoliosis in children, but they don't generally prevent or alleviate low back pain.

A brace might be effective for acute pain in the short term, but it might not. Short-term bracing with a Velcro stretch corset, though, has little downside, and so I don't oppose it. It's in the long term that bracing goes wrong.

For starters, if your spine is immobilized, or its movement is restricted, you don't use the muscles, ligaments, and tendons around your spine. If you don't use them, they get deconditioned. Since you (hopefully) just finished the chapter on exercise, you already know that strong, conditioned muscles can help relieve back pain. It's safe to conclude that weak, deconditioned muscles are unlikely to do you any good and may make your pain worse. Your bones also lose by being exempted from daily wear and tear. Stress is good for bones, and bones that aren't stressed are at risk for osteoporosis.

The comfort and convenience of the brace are also issues. If it's uncomfortable to wear, or difficult to get in and out of, it can raise stress levels at a time when decreasing stress and increasing comfort are important to recovery. If it doesn't fit right, and rubs against your skin, it can cause sores or abrasions. Mental and physical irritation won't help back pain.

On the opposite end of brace problems is dependency. I've seen patients who wore braces for so long that they became dependent on them—physically, mentally, or both. The brace eventually became an extension of themselves, and they had to be weaned off it.

CASE STUDY

MARYBETH was twelve years old when she first came to me with scoliosis serious enough to require a brace. At first, she was resistant to the idea of a brace—most kids are—but her parents and I convinced her to try it. It worked. The curvature of her spine didn't change, and the brace helped her avoid the necessity of surgery. After three years, we started to wean her off it by having her wear it for fewer hours every day. She had no trouble going through the day without it,

but she wanted to continue to wear it at night, partly because she was accustomed to sleeping that way, and partly
because she was afraid her scoliosis would worsen if she
stopped bracing. Eventually, I made a contract with her. I
would let her lessen her dependence in her own way over
the course of two months, but, when those two months
were over, I would take the brace. She did, and I did, and
she's doing fine.

There are situations when a brace is thought to be helpful, but
they are few and specific:

scoliosis in children and adolescents
fractures (osteoporotic or traumatic)
post–fusion surgery

Other than for those situations, there is only one kind of
brace I can recommend: Velcro stretch supports for heavy la-
borers. If you're loading boxes or hauling lumber or lifting produce, you may be able to reduce the intensity and frequency of
back pain episodes by wearing one of those (admittedly unat-
tractive) black belts while you work. Not all research supports
the effectiveness of the belts, but they won't do you harm.
Other than that, I recommend against the long-term use of any
brace for back pain. No benefits have been firmly established,
and I've seen too many patients with too many problems to
take the risk.

BED REST

In the last thirty years, prolonged bed rest has gone from being the treatment of choice for many back ailments to being
Spine Enemy Number One. For an acute episode of pain, or for

recovery from a surgical procedure, you may need to spend two to three days in bed. Beyond that, though, you need to be up and, if not running, at least walking.

If your back problem is so painful that you can't get out of bed, you need to see a doctor who'll help you get back on your feet. Two things will go wrong if you don't: your back won't get better and the rest of you will get worse. For starters, your muscles will atrophy, which means they won't be able to support you properly when you do stand up. Muscles also tend to tighten and spasm when you don't use them (think about the last long flight you took). If that's not enough to scare you upright, there's also the chance of a blood clot in your legs and the risk of pneumonia and bedsores, particularly in the elderly.

But the biggest problem with bed rest is that it doesn't work. Study after study has shown that getting out of bed is the best bet for back pain.

While you are trying different alternative treatments, there is a good chance that your doctor will recommend some type of medication. Medication can be combined with any of the alternative treatments. In the next chapter, I discuss the role of medication in your treatment and what to expect from it.

ENDNOTES

i M. W. van Tulder, et al., "The Effectiveness of Acupuncture in the Management of Acute and Chronic Low Back Pain: A Systematic Review Within the Framework of the Cochrane Collaboration Back Review Group," *Spine* 24, no. 11 (1999), pp. 1113–23.

ii E. Manheimer, et al., "Meta-Analysis: Acupuncture for Low Back Pain," *Annals of Internal Medicine* 142 (2005), pp. 651–63.

iii D. M. Eisenberg, et al., "Trends in Alternative Medicine Use in the United States, 1990–1997: Results of a Follow-up National Survey," *Journal of the American Medical Association* 280, no. 18 (1998), pp. 1569–75.

iv W. J. Assendelft, et al., "Spinal Manipulative Therapy for Low Back Pain: A Meta-Analysis of Effectiveness Relative to Other Therapies," *Annals of Internal Medicine* 138 (2003), pp. 871–81.

v T. Tullberg, et al., "Manipulation Does Not Alter the Position of the Sacroiliac Joint: A Roentgen Stereophotogrammetric Analysis," *Spine* 23, no. 10 (1998), pp. 1124–28.

vi E. L. Hurwitz, et al., "Second Prize: The Effectiveness of Physical Modalities Among Patients With Low Back Pain Randomized to Chiropractic Care: Findings from the UCLA Low Back Pain Study," *Journal of Manipulative and Physiological Therapeutics* 25, no. 1 (2002), pp. 10–20.

vii E. L. Hurwitz, et al., "Manipulation and Mobilization of the Cervical Spine: A Systematic Review of the Literature," *Spine* 21, no. 15 (1996), pp. 1746–59.

Chapter 10

MEDICATIONS

Pain is personal. That's what makes treating it difficult. If I were to prescribe medication for cholesterol, or blood pressure, or eczema, I could assess the condition and measure the results. With pain, though, I can do neither. I rely on my patients to tell me both how bad the pain is and how significant the relief is. If pain medication didn't have a downside, that wouldn't be so hard. More would be better. But all—let me repeat, all—medications have a downside, and more is more dangerous. Obviously, though, they also have an upside. For many patients with back pain, the right pain medication can make the difference between having surgery and not having it.

In all the years I've been practicing medicine, I've never worked with a patient who hasn't tried pain medication at some point. It's part of just about every treatment regimen for back pain, from physical therapy to fusion surgery. And it's a critical part. Pain can be devastating. It can be the root of physical, emotional, economic, and social damage, both for patients in pain and the people around them. Although it's invisible and unmeasurable, pain can ruin lives as surely as accidents or diseases.

Despite their importance in treating back pain, I've found that the ins and outs of pain medications are poorly understood by most patients, who don't know an NSAID from an opiate. This chapter will make sure that you're not one of those patients. It will give you the pluses and minuses of all the major players in the pain medication field, and help you help your doctor medicate your pain while keeping side effects to a minimum.

Before I go into specific medications, I want to cover a couple of general drug-related issues that apply to everything on this list.

Generic or name brand? Some patients (and some doctors) prefer the name-brand version of some medications, but there's no evidence that the big brands are any more effective than the generics. When there's a choice, I generally go generic.

What's the dose? Toxicologists have a saying: the dose is the poison. You can kill yourself with just about anything, including water, if you ingest enough of it. All of the medications in this chapter are safe at one dose and unsafe at another. Always follow directions, whether they're on the medicine's label (if it's over-the-counter) or on your doctor's prescription.

How often do I take them? No more often than the label says, whether it's a prescription or over-the-counter medication. You do have options, though. Some medications are prescribed "as needed" and others are taken at regular intervals. If you have trouble remembering to take pills, you may want to consider a medication that you only have to take once a day, or a slow-release version of a medication that you'd ordinarily have to take more than once a day.

Is it contraindicated? "Contraindicated" means that there is some condition, specific to you, that makes taking a particular drug a riskier-than-normal proposition. It could be because you have a disease or condition that the drug is bad for, or because you're taking other medications with which the drug doesn't mix well. If you have an ulcer, for example, you shouldn't be on anti-inflammatories, because they can make your ulcer bleed. The key to avoiding contraindicated medications is full disclosure. Tell your doctor about any medical conditions you have, and all medications you take, including vitamins and herbal supplements.

Will my pain go away? Usually not completely. Don't go into this thinking that there's a pill out there that will magically give you a pain-free existence. The goal of pain medication is to lessen pain to the point that you can handle it.

Can I mix and match? It's tempting to try several different pain medications with several different mechanisms in the hope of relieving pain more thoroughly. And it sometimes works well. Often, though, it's a bad idea. Some medications interact, and some combinations can be downright dangerous. Some medications also shouldn't be combined with alcohol, and you should never use street drugs when you're on any medication. Mixing and matching can work, but leave it to the professionals. Specifically, leave it to one professional. Get your pain medications from one, and only one, doctor. If you go to more than one, it's possible to get prescriptions that shouldn't go together.

Does it have to be a pill? No, although pills are by far the most common delivery mechanism. If you have trouble swallowing pills, you may want to consider a medication that comes in a liquid form, like codeine. Some medications (like opiates) also come in transdermal patches. You put the patch on your skin and get a constant flow of medication for several days. One anti-inflammatory (indomethacin) comes as a suppository. If you're hospitalized, and put on opiates, you may get an injection or an intravenous pump so you can control the dose yourself; this method is called patient-controlled anesthesia (PCA).

Can I drive? You can usually drive and do every other daily activity when you're on pain medication, although it makes sense to use caution. Don't drive when you're on narcotics, and talk to your doctor if you have any questions.

These questions, and this chapter, only scratch the surface of the issue of medication. There are too many choices, and too many considerations for each choice, for me to be able to give you a comprehensive overview. What's covered here are the most important medications, the most important issues, the most serious side effects, and the most common contraindications. But remember that all medications have side effects, can cause allergies, and can interact with other medications. It is outside the scope of this book to cover them all. If you have any medical condition, advise your doctor. Pay attention to the dose and frequency of the medication. Of course, read the product information that comes with your medication. For complete information on any medication you're taking or considering, consult with your doctor. You can also get information on the Internet site of the National Institutes of Health, www.nlm.nih.gov/medlineplus.

ACETAMINOPHEN

Good old Tylenol. Chances are it's in your medicine cabinet already. It is one of the most reliable, safest analgesics (the technical term for pain relievers) we've got. Tylenol is available generically almost everywhere, and it's often my first choice for treating mild to moderate back pain.

There are several theories of how acetaminophen works, and why it works so well, but I'm going to spare you the chemistry lesson because nobody's exactly sure. Suffice it to say that almost everyone who takes it experiences at least some pain relief.

I'm going to make an exception to my prohibition against

mixing and matching medications at home. Acetaminophen combines very well with NSAIDs (see page 159). I've had many patients who don't respond particularly well to either one but get almost complete relief from the combination.

On the downside, the biggest risk of acetaminophen is liver damage, so it's important to keep track of how much you're taking. Liver toxicity can begin at 10–15 grams in one dose, and 20–25 grams can be fatal. As you add up your daily milligrams, make sure you check the labels of all the medications you're taking. One Extra Strength Tylenol is 500 milligrams (a half a gram), but acetaminophen isn't just in things labeled Tylenol. It sneaks into a lot of products where you might not expect it, such as:

cold and flu medication
Vicodin
Percocet
Darvocet

(The suffix -cet usually means that there's acetaminophen in a medication, although the absence of that suffix doesn't mean it doesn't have acetaminophen.)

To make it harder, acetaminophen is sold under different names in different countries. If you've got back pain in Belgium, look for Lemgrip. In Singapore, it's Napa. Closer to home, it's Panadol or Feverall or Abenol or Tempra. Wherever you are, check the fine print. Somewhere on the label it'll say acetaminophen.

Contraindications: Although acetaminophen is one of the safest pain medications, there are conditions that put you at higher risk for side effects. If you have any of these, make sure you tell your doctor before you embark on a pain medication regimen:

anemia

alcoholism

infection (because acetaminophen will mask the symptoms)

kidney or liver disease

hepatitis

phenylketonuria (It's a rare genetic disease; if you have it, you
know.)

allergic reaction to acetaminophen, aspirin, or NSAIDs

ASPIRIN

Whatever happened to "take two aspirins and call me in the
morning"? Pain relief has improved, that's what. Don't get me
wrong—aspirin is amazing stuff. It's a blood thinner, and taken
regularly it can help fight heart disease, stroke, and other conditions. But don't get the idea that because it's been around forever
and we've all taken it since childhood that it's the safest choice
for back pain. It's not a potent pain reliever and the long-term
use of doses high enough to treat serious pain is too risky for aspirin to be a good choice for back pain management; the blood-
thinning effect can result in stomach ulcers and internal bleeding.
I don't recommend aspirin for back pain.

NONSTEROIDAL ANTI-INFLAMMATORY
DRUGS (NSAIDS)

They're the most widely used pain medication in existence, val-
ued for their reliable effectiveness. They all have side effects, and
those side effects are common, but they can generally be managed

by fitting the right medication at the right dose with the right person.

As their name implies, NSAIDs fight pain by fighting inflammation, which is often the source of pain. Most back pain is rooted in inflammation, and so NSAIDs are very useful. One of the reasons I use NSAIDS is that they actually tackle the source of the problem rather than simply masking the pain.

There are different kinds of NSAIDs, and in order to choose the right kind you have to understand how they work. So this time I'm afraid you're going to have to sit through the chemistry lesson.

NSAIDs work by blocking the body's production of a group of chemicals called prostaglandins, which are produced in many of your organs and set off the production of a cascade of chemicals that are irritants and are an integral part of pain. Your body produces them by taking a chemical called arachidonic acid and converting it with an enzyme called cyclooxygenase. Before you throw up your hands at all the unpronounceable names, let me make a bet with you—I'll bet you've heard of COX inhibitors. Yes? I thought so. Well, that's where all this comes together. COX stands for cyclooxygenase, the enzyme that is responsible for converting arachidonic acid to prostaglandins. No COX, no conversion. No conversion, no prostaglandins. No prostaglandins, no pain. Or at least less pain.

There are two kinds of COX. COX-1 is body-wide, and COX-2 is found mostly in injured or inflamed tissue. Most NSAIDs block both kinds of COX; those are the nonselective NSAIDs. Some, though, block only COX-2; those are the newer, selective kind, and they have several advantages. Prostaglandins, particularly the COX-1 kind, don't just exist to cause pain. They have other functions in the body (such as blood clotting), and blocking them can cause ulcers and bleeding. By blocking only COX-2, selective NSAIDs minimize that danger. The selective NSAIDs are expensive, and they're only available by prescription, but if you have a history of ulcers or bleeding problems, you and your doctor may want to consider them.

The COX-2 medications have gotten a lot of attention since the withdrawal of Vioxx (rofecoxib) from the market. Some 20 million Americans took Vioxx before safety concerns about cardiovascular risks (including heart attack and stroke) forced its withdrawal. Another COX-2 NSAID, Bextra (valdecoxib), was subsequently withdrawn for similar reasons. Celebrex (celecoxib) is the only COX-2 selective NSAID left on the market, and it's available only by prescription. The FDA has asked that all prescription NSAIDS have a highlighted, boxed warning about the possibility of increased risk of cardiovascular events and potentially life-threatening gastrointestinal bleeding, and research is under way to determine the long-term safety of these NSAIDS. Should you take them? There's no definitive answer; I think the risk-benefit equation varies by individual. If you're considering them, talk to your doctor.

Because taking NSAIDs can promote bleeding, you may have to stop taking them a week or more before any invasive procedure. It's particularly important for fusion surgery, since the drugs can interfere with the bone's ability to regenerate. If you're getting a fusion, you should discontinue NSAIDs well before the procedure, and stay off them until your fusion has healed.

Aside from ulcers and bleeding, the primary side effects of NSAIDs are stomach pain and nausea, but the likelihood is small. There is also the chance of damage to other organs, which is why patients with organ-related conditions should only take

NSAIDs under a doctor's care. And, as with all medications, pay attention to the dose and don't take more than is prescribed or indicated on the label.

Here's a partial list of the different types of NSAIDs. New versions are in development, though, so your doctor may recommend one that's unfamiliar. (Some of the prescription nonselective NSAIDs come in generic versions. If that's important, mention it to your doctor.)

PRESCRIPTION NONSELECTIVE

Generic Name	Brand Name
Diclofenac	Voltaren
Diflunisal	Dolobid
Etodolac	Lodine
Fenoprofen	Nalfon
Flurbiprofen	Ansaid
Indomethacin	Indocin
Ketoprofen	Orudis
Ketorolac	Toradol
Meclofenamate	Meclomen
Mefenamic acid	Ponstel
Meloxicam	Mobic
Nabumetone	Relafen
Oxaprozin	Daypro
Piroxicam	Feldene
Sulindac	Clinoril
Tolmetin	Tolectin

PRESCRIPTION COX-2

Generic Name	Brand Name
Celecoxib	Celebrex

OVER-THE-COUNTER

Generic Name	Brand Name
Ibuprofen	Advil, Motrin
Naproxen	Aleve

Although their mechanism is similar, NSAIDs are all a little different from each other. I've seen patients try three or four with no success, and then do well on the fourth or fifth. Each person reacts a little differently to each medication, and it's worth trying several to find the one that works best. You'll get a good idea of an NSAID's effectiveness after taking it for two to three days. If it's not working, move on to the next.

Contraindications: NSAIDs, particularly the selective kind, are quite safe. These are some of the conditions that might put you at higher risk:

kidney, liver or cardiac disease
history of ulcers
diabetes
allergies to NSAIDs or aspirin

There are also medications that might interact with NSAIDs, so make sure to tell your doctor if you are taking any medication, and especially any of these:

other NSAIDs
aspirin
blood thinners (Coumadin, Plavix)
steroids (prednisone)
herbal supplements
antihypertensive medications
chemotherapy medications
psychotropic medications
immunosuppressive medications

OPIATES

It sounds like opium, and for good reason. All the opiates (also known as opioids) are related, and they all come from the same kind of opium-producing poppy. Or at least they did originally—now we can make them synthetically. When we talk about narcotics, we're generally, but not always, talking about opiates. This group includes a lot of powerful drugs. Some of them, like morphine and codeine, are useful in treating serious pain. Others, like heroin, don't have clinical use. I'm not here to lecture you, but I strongly advise you not to even think about using any street drug for pain relief.

Opiates work by binding themselves to the opioid receptors, which is where pain signals are received. If they're blocked, your brain can't receive the pain signal and you can't feel the pain. Unlike NSAIDs, opiates don't tackle the source of the pain; they only hide it from your brain.

If you've been watching too many old movies, and you have visions of getting addicted to opium, losing all interest in life and spending all your hours in a smoky opium den, you shouldn't worry too much. It is possible to get addicted to opiates, but it's not nearly as common as you may think. If you work closely with your doctor, and follow directions, you're unlikely to get addicted to opiates. If, however, you start doing things like filling more and more prescriptions, or taking higher and higher doses, you could be developing a tolerance, a situation in which your body requires more and more medication for the same response. Anyone who uses opiates for extended periods may develop a tolerance for them. After a while, you'll find that they don't work as well, and you have to increase the dose or the frequency to get the same level of pain relief. Work closely with your doctor to make any adjustments to your medication.

Dependence is another concern when taking opiates. Whereas an addiction is characterized by a lack of control over the use of a substance, a dependence simply means that you'll have some withdrawal symptoms if you stop or significantly reduce the dose suddenly. Opiates often cause dependence, and if you've been using them for some time you should anticipate it. When it's time to go off them, your doctor will help you wean yourself off slowly.

Like other types of pain medication, opiates differ. Some are better for acute pain, such as that from a fracture or other trauma. Others are better for chronic pain. Different doctors have different preferences. Here are some common opiates used for pain:

GENERIC	BRAND NAME
Codeine	Codeine
Oxycodone	Oxycontin
Hydrocodone	Lortab
Propoxyphene	Darvon
Pentazocine	Talwin
Tramadol	Ultram
Hydromorphone	Dilaudid
Morphine	Roxanol

Many opiates are combined by pharmaceutical firms with acetominophen. The combination makes for a potentiated effect. Some common combinations include:

BRAND NAME	MEDICATIONS INSIDE
Ultracet	tramadol + acetominophen
Norco/Lorcet	hydrocodone + acetominophen
Tylenol #3	codeine + acetominophen
Tylox, Roxicet, Percocet	oxycodone + acetominophen
Darvocet, Wygesic, Propacet	propoxyphene + acetominophen

Most of the side effects of opiates are a result of the fact that they are depressants, and they slow down your whole system. One commonly overlooked side effect is constipation; I've had patients whose bowels slowed to a crawl. Other common side effects are fatigue, nausea, and lack of concentration. Less common side effects are mood changes, loss of appetite, itchiness, urinary hesitancy, sexual dysfunction, headaches, sleep difficulty, chest pain, and headaches. If you experience any of these, let your doctor know. Often, you can change the medicine or the dose (or both) and still get the pain relief without the unpleasant side effects.

Contraindications: There are many reasons not to use opiates, and they're different for each medication. If you have any other medical problem, make sure you tell your doctor before you take any narcotic.

MUSCLE RELAXANTS

You probably think muscle relaxants work to relieve LBP by relaxing the muscles, but the truth is that we don't have a good understanding of how they work. They do indeed help with muscle spasms, which are a common source of back pain, but they probably work in the brain and spinal cord, and not directly in the muscle. The role of muscle spasm as a cause of back pain itself remains controversial. Nevertheless, muscle relaxants are commonly used for both acute and chronic low back pain. And they seem to work. At least a little.

A review of the most recent studies shows muscle relaxants to be better than placebo, and there may be an added benefit when they are used in conjunction with NSAIDs. We are still not sure if they are more effective than analgesics or NSAIDs. The beneficial effects of treatment with muscle relaxants does not last long—at best, a couple of weeks. Beyond that, long-term use has not been shown to have any beneficial effect. Though there are many different muscle relaxants to choose from, it doesn't seem to matter which one you pick; they all seem to perform with only moderate results.[i]

To summarize, if muscle relaxants work for either acute or chronic LBP, they are probably best for short-term use. They are also used to reduce spasticity in cerebral palsy, multiple sclerosis, spinal cord injury, and other spasm-related conditions.

Here are some common muscle relaxants:

NONBENZODIAZEPINES

Brand Name	Generic Name
Flexeril	cyclobenzaprine
Skelaxin	metaxalone
Robaxin	methocarbamol
Soma	carisoprodol
Norflex	orphenadrine
Zanaflex	tizanidine

ANTISPASTICITY MEDICATIONS
Baclofen
Dantrolene sodium

BENZODIAZEPINES

Brand Name	Generic Name
Valium	diazepam

The adverse effects of muscle relaxants warrant consideration and are often the limiting factor in their use. They include dizziness, drowsiness, and impaired balance. Most people who take muscle relaxants experience at least one of these. If you have any pre-existing medical condition or an organ-related disease, you should discuss this further with your physician before taking these drugs.

ANTIDEPRESSANTS

Wait. What are antidepressants doing in the chapter on pain medication? Or in a book on spine surgery, for that matter? It turns out that antidepressants (ADs) can help treat chronic pain. This is particularly true of one group of ADs—the tricyclics (the selective serotonin uptake inhibitors, or SSRIs, don't work as well). Nobody knows why ADs work for pain. Doctors took note when some of their patients who took the tricyclic ADs for depression reported chronic pain relief as a side effect, and pretty soon they started prescribing them for pain. If you suffer from anxiety or depression, both of which can reduce your pain threshold, ADs may be particularly beneficial. Be aware that the benefits may take as long as two weeks to kick in, so give them time, and don't expect to use them for acute pain.

The most common side effects of ADs are sleepiness, dry mouth, and palpitation. Some patients also experience sexual dysfunction. If you have prostate problems, cardiac arrhythmias, glaucoma, hypotension, or severe constipation, or take any number of other medications, you shouldn't take antidepressants.

ANTISEIZURE MEDICATIONS

Although antiseizure medications haven't been FDA-approved for pain relief, they are sometimes effective, and their prescription is common. They are used for nerve and specifically radicular symptoms, such as sciatica. They have not been shown to help with acute or chronic low back pain. Nobody knows exactly why they work, but it's believed that whatever mechanism causes nerves to be irritable in seizures may be related to pain in sciatica. In the back realm, antiseizure medications can help only radicular and neuropathic pain.

STEROIDS

Steroids are powerful fighters of inflammation and swelling, and can therefore help fight inflammation-related pain. They're not the same as the anabolic steroids you've read about athletes taking, but they're related. The steroids we use for pain management are very powerful anti-inflammatories. There are two kinds: oral and locally injected. I cover injectable steroids in chapter 11. Oral steroids are occasionally prescribed for severe sciatica from a herniated disc, but there's no compelling evidence that they work.

The goals of pain medication are to reduce pain, enhance quality of life, and increase the ability to function, all while minimizing the risk of adverse effects. If the site of pain can be localized to a particular nerve or structure, medication can be injected directly into the site. The following chapter covers spinal injections, which may be an adjunct to relieving your pain with oral medication.

ENDNOTE

i M. W. van Tulder, et al., "Muscle Relaxants for Nonspecific Low Back Pain: A Systematic Review Within the Framework of the Cochrane Collaboration," *Spine* 28, no. 17 (2003), pp. 1978–92.

Chapter 11

SPINAL INJECTIONS

Yes, spinal injections require a needle to be inserted into your spine. If your first thought is "Ouch!" you're not alone. When I talk to patients about spinal injections, I can see their faces contort at the very thought of it. Once I assure them that we can minimize the pain of the injection by applying a local anesthetic, and *then* the big needle into the spine, we can get down to business.

There are two kinds of spinal injections: diagnostic and therapeutic. The diagnostic kind do exactly what you'd expect: help your doctor figure out where the problem is (or isn't). The therapeutic kind blocks pain. By rights, diagnostic injections should be in the chapter on testing, but since they're usually just a variation of therapeutic injections, and so often done in conjunction with them, I'm grouping them all together here.

Diagnostic and therapeutic injections work on a very simple principle. Diagnostically, if we numb a specific site on your spine and your pain stops, there's a good chance the site is causing the pain and we can narrow down a diagnosis. Therapeutically, if we can stop the swelling in an inflamed site on your spine and your pain stops—your pain stops! And isn't that what you went to the doctor for in the first place?

The key difference between diagnostic and therapeutic injections is what gets injected. For diagnosis, we use a short-acting numbing medication like the kind you get at the dentist. The numbing effect of these kinds of medications lasts eight hours at the longest. That's not long if you're thinking in terms of pain relief, but it's certainly long enough for diagnosis.

> **Your spinal injection: diagnosis, treatment, or both?** Spinal injections are used to either diagnose or treat pain. Sometimes they are done together. Be sure to understand the difference between these two objectives *before* getting your injection.

For treating pain, we inject much longer-acting steroids. Their anti-inflammatory properties make them potent local pain fighters, and although the steroids themselves are absorbed by the body in just a couple of days, the relief can last much longer, sometimes forever—I've had patients who got one injection and never experienced pain again. Don't expect permanence, though. Results vary markedly. I've had patients postpone surgery for years, or even indefinitely, because therapeutic injections work so well for them, and I've also had patients who aren't so fortunate. Not all pain responds to injections, and symptoms other than pain almost never respond. If you have numbness, tingling, weakness, or other nerve-related symptoms, don't expect injections to make them go away.

The tricky part of spinal injections is knowing where to inject them. Choosing the target site is a kind of mix-and-match process. If the pain is localized to the back, I might target an irritated tendon, a facet joint, or even the sacroiliac joint. If the pain is radicular, an inflamed nerve is the target. Matching the site to the pain is not always as easy as it sounds. It's probably clear to you by now that the nature of pain and the nature of backs are such that the match is often not nearly as clear as we'd like it to be. When injections don't work, and they sometimes don't, it can be because there's a mismatch between pain and site. It's also possible, though, that the site is causing the pain but the pain isn't alleviated by the injection.

For some patients, and for some pain, injections are a low-risk, viable alternative to surgery. Elderly patients, particularly, for whom surgery may be a riskier proposition, are good candidates for pain management by injection. Unless there's a compelling reason to operate, I'm happy to work closely with patients to manage their pain this way. Your surgeon may refer you to a pain specialist for pain management with injections. There's very little literature on how patients do with frequent injections over a long period of time, and the decision to inject or not to inject generally has more to do with a doctor's preference than any concrete risks or benefits.

What we know for sure is that injections don't cure; they won't fix your facet joints or un-herniate your disc. They're a pain management tool, but a powerful one.

TYPES OF INJECTIONS

This chapter covers the most common spinal injections, but the following list isn't exhaustive. There are many different back-related injections that are done rarely and in very specific circumstances. If you're getting one of them, make sure you talk to your doctor about what it's going to do for you, and what its

risks are. Most injections, though, fall into one of these categories:

INJECTION	TARGET
epidural steroid injections	nerves in the spinal canal
trigger point injections	tendons and muscles
facet joint injections	facet joint and surrounding nerves
sacroiliac joint injections	sacroiliac joint
selective nerve root block	isolated nerve root

Most injections can be either diagnostic or therapeutic, but I
cover two exceptions in this book. The first is the myelogram,
which is only diagnostic, and is covered in the testing chapter on
page 80. The second is the epidural steroid injection, which is
only therapeutic. Let's start with that.

EPIDURAL STEROID INJECTIONS

If you or someone you know has ever had a baby, chances are
you know about epidural injections. When an epidural is used in
anesthesia, a numbing medicine is injected directly into the
epidural space, where it bathes the spinal nerves. The result is
that while the medicine is working, you don't feel the lower part
of the body—an effect that has obvious implications for child-
birth. An epidural steroid injection works the same way, except
that what's injected is an anti-inflammatory steroid. Steroids
have the potential to reduce swelling and inflammation of
nerves. If that's not what's causing your pain, the injection probably won't work.

Epidural steroid injections can be very effective for some kinds
of pain, and completely ineffective for others. Because they're
aimed at nerves, they can only reliably help with nerve-related,
radicular pain. Pain from a herniated disc responds best, but

stenosis patients may also benefit. For herniated discs, epidural injections are most effective when they're done within six weeks of the onset of pain. For stenosis, if they work at all, the timing doesn't seem to matter.

If your pain is primarily back pain, don't expect epidural steroids to help. Ditto if you've been diagnosed with a degenerated disc or internal disc disruption. And if there's any chance that your pain is being caused by a tumor, a fracture, or an infection, you shouldn't even consider injections; you need treatment of the cause, not the pain.

Even if your pain is radicular, and your diagnosis is stenosis or herniation, injections aren't foolproof; they work about 60–70 percent of the time. That's pretty good, though, especially when the alternative is surgery.

The details of the procedure are straightforward. The doctor injects steroids into the epidural space. Most of the time, she'll do it by inserting a needle in the middle of the back directly into the spinal canal. That's called a translaminar injection, because the needle goes in between the laminae of two adjacent vertebrae (see illustration). Occasionally, she'll choose to feed a catheter into the spinal canal from the tailbone in a procedure called a caudal injection. Either way, she may or may not use a fluoroscope, a kind of X-ray that can help position the needle.

Although epidural injections don't fix the underlying problem, by alleviating pain they buy time. Often, pain from stenosis or a herniated disc eventually goes away by itself, but many patients can't wait it out—especially since there's no guarantee it will stop.

TRIGGER POINT INJECTIONS

A trigger point injection is a shot of steroids directly into the muscle or tendon that hurts. On page 50 I mentioned myofascial pain, which is localized muscle or tendon pain that doesn't

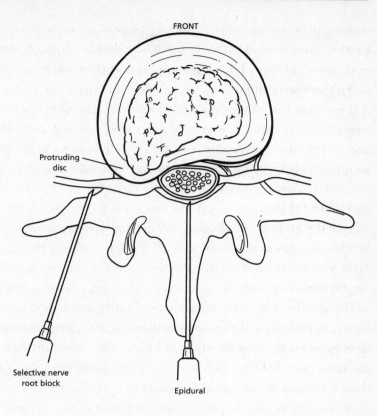

FRONT

Protruding
disc

Selective nerve
root block

Epidural

The two most common nerve injections: In an epidural injection (midline needle), the tip of the needle is inside the spinal canal, injecting steroids around all of the nerves in the vicinity. In a selective nerve root block (needle to the side), the needle is outside the spinal canal and only one nerve is treated. Although shown together, these procedures are not usually performed together.

involve the spine. A trigger point injection is the only treatment in this book specifically for myofascial pain, although other treatments for spine-related pain may also help alleviate it.

Trigger point injections are simple and easy to perform. They're essentially risk-free and any doctor can do them in his office. The downside is that they don't work all that well. They may help you and they may not, but if you have a localized pain in the soft tissue in your back, they may be worth trying.

FACET JOINT INJECTIONS

These are injections into the facet joint that can affect both the joint itself and the microscopic nerves that provide sensation to it. (Don't confuse these nerves with the spinal nerves that cause radicular pain.) Painful facet joints are usually caused by arthritis, which is caused by worn-down cartilage, bone spurs, or cysts, and if a diagnostic injection establishes that a facet joint is indeed the cause of your pain, then your doctor can inject longer-acting steroids for a therapeutic effect. The injection can be made directly into the joint itself, or just outside the joint if the goal is to treat the surrounding nerves.

When a facet joint is the problem, it causes back pain, not leg pain, and so facet joint injections can only help if your pain is in the back. It's the facet itself that hurts, and not the spinal nerves that run close by.

SACROILIAC JOINT INJECTIONS

These are very similar to the facet joint injections, but done in the sacroiliac joint. They aren't as common, though, because the sacroiliac joint is only rarely isolated as the source of pain. (The SI joint and problems with it are described on page 117.)

SELECTIVE NERVE ROOT BLOCK

A selective nerve root block, also called a foraminal or trans-foraminal injection, is aimed specifically at one nerve. If your doctor identifies a particular nerve that she thinks is causing your pain, she'll numb it with a selective nerve root block to see whether the pain stops (that's diagnostic). If the pain does stop, she can then inject a steroid to treat the pain (that's therapeutic).

Because this is an injection into one nerve and one nerve only, accurate placement of the needle is critical (see illustration on page 175). That's why selective nerve root blocks are always done with a fluoroscope or CT scan.

RISKS OF INJECTIONS

There aren't very many. There's a very small risk of the usual problems you can have with any kind of injection—infection, hematoma, nerve injury, spinal fluid leak. But it's reasonable to think of these procedures as safe.

The risk my patients worry about is barely a risk at all: steroids. They hear the word, and they think of all those baseball players and teenagers doing horrible things to their bodies in the pursuit of big muscles. But the steroids we use in injections aren't the anabolic steroids that cast a shadow over professional sports and give rise to congressional hearings. If you have an injection, your face won't puff up, you won't get cataracts or osteoporosis or diabetes. Of course, you also won't set any home run records.

No matter what kind of injection you get, and no matter how small the risks, the possibility of complications does go up if your doctor is inexperienced. Some injections are difficult to get just right, and practice helps a lot. Don't hesitate to ask how often, and how recently, your doctor has given them.

The treatments you've read about so far, from exercise to

GOING UNDER THE KNIFE

Surgical Procedures

Chapter 12

LUMBAR LAMINECTOMY

The longest section of this book is the one on surgical procedures—the very procedures I wrote the book to help you avoid. The reason it's the longest is because deciding whether to get surgery is the most difficult decision back pain patients face, and you need to know a lot to make an educated decision. I'm going to start with a procedure that has a proven track record—lumbar laminectomy. It is the most commonly performed spine surgery in the United States, and a good place to start your surgical education. To understand the procedure, you might first need a refresher course on vertebral structure. The lamina is the part of the vertebra that's at the base of the bumps that run down your back. Each vertebra has two laminae, one on each side. Because of their position, the laminae are the easiest place for your surgeon to gain access to the nerves in your spine. When it comes to surgery, the lamina acts as a kind of garage door to the spinal canal, the tube running from your head to your tailbone through which the spinal cord and nerves run. When that tube gets narrowed by a condition like a herniated disc or spinal stenosis, the nerves may be compressed. The way your surgeon gets in to remove whatever is compressing the nerves is through the lamina. Removing some or all of it opens the garage door and gives your surgeon access to the spinal canal.

THE VARIETIES OF LAMINECTOMY

Laminectomy is a generic category that really encompasses two different procedures: laminectomy proper, and laminotomy. The suffixes give you a clue to the difference: -ectomy means that you're removing something, and -otomy means that you're cutting

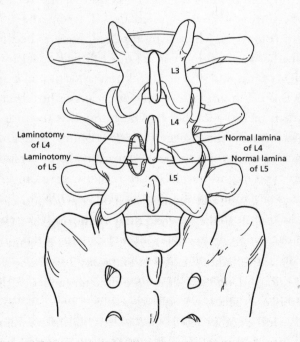

Laminotomy of L4
Laminotomy of L5

L3
L4
L5

Normal lamina of L4
Normal lamina of L5

A one-sided laminotomy, creating a small window in the lamina above and the same in the lamina below. Note the preserved remaining lamina (on the right side) and spinous process.

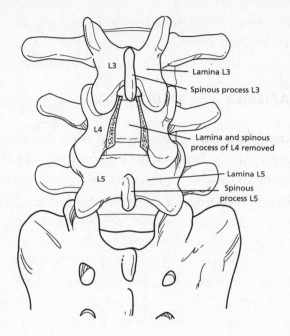

L3

Lamina L3

Spinous process L3

L4

Lamina and spinous
process of L4 removed

L5

Lamina L5

Spinous
process L5

A complete laminectomy of the entire L4 lamina and spinous process.

into it. You're undoubtedly familiar with other procedures that use those suffixes, such as the appendectomy (removing the appendix) or tonsillectomy (removing the tonsil). Likewise, a laminectomy removes the entire lamina, and a laminotomy only removes part (see illustrations). Don't get hung up on the terminology, though; some doctors use the terms interchangeably.

There are lots of other words used to describe different kinds of laminectomies, and most are self-explanatory. A partial laminectomy is the same as a laminotomy. A one-sided laminotomy takes out a piece of the lamina on one side. A complete laminectomy takes out the entire lamina on both sides, as well as the spinous process in between (which means you end up with a flat spot on your back where the bump used to be). A multilevel laminectomy is a complete laminectomy on two or more vertebrae. You'll also see laminectomy paired with decompression. "Decompression" just means taking pressure off the nerves, which, with very few exceptions, is the only reason to do a laminectomy.

Regardless of what he calls the procedure, your surgeon will remove just enough of the bone to give him access to the spinal canal to do what he has to do, and the nature and severity of your condition will determine just how much that is. If the problem is localized and specific (such as a herniated disc), your surgeon may be able to remove the material pressing on your spinal nerves through a very small opening in the lamina. If the problem is more extensive (such as spinal stenosis), your surgeon may have to remove the whole lamina for easier access. Technically, the first procedure is a laminotomy and the second a laminectomy, but in this book I use "laminectomy" generically unless the distinction is important.

WHY A LAMINECTOMY?

Laminectomies and laminotomies are a little different from most other operations that end in -ectomy or -otomy. Usually, the reason to take something out is that it's causing a problem. The lamina, though, is rarely the problem. The lamina is simply bone that blocks your surgeon's access to the problem, and it has to be taken out to get there.

The problem is something—anything—that narrows the spinal canal. Anything that generates material that's not supposed to be there (such as a tumor) or displaces material that's supposed to be somewhere else (such as a herniated disc or a fracture) can end up depositing something in the spinal canal that houses the cauda equina and the spinal nerves. Whatever it is that gets in there shouldn't be there, and if it severely presses on a nerve, you may need to get it out.

The two most common conditions that are treated with a laminectomy are herniated discs and spinal stenosis. For a herniated disc, the procedure most commonly performed is called a microdiscectomy, or discectomy for short. Your surgeon uses a microscope or special magnifying glasses called loupes to get a better view of what is a very small space. He opens up a small part of the garage door (lamina) and removes the material that has oozed out of the disc (he doesn't remove the whole disc, just the escaped part). For stenosis, a laminectomy is usually required, since he needs better access to remove all of the material that has intruded into the epidural space. In doing the decompression, he relieves the pressure on the nerves and, hopefully, stops the pain in your legs.

And now we get to the single most important point I want you to understand about laminectomies. They fix leg pain, not back pain. The goal of a laminectomy is simple and straightforward: to remove pressure on a nerve. Therefore, the only kind of pain a laminectomy can fix is the kind that results from nerve pressure. That's radicular pain (for a herniated disc) or neurogenic claudication pain (for spinal stenosis).

> **Laminectomies are for leg pain.** Removing the lamina allows your surgeon access to the spinal canal where he can relieve pressure on a compressed nerve. Pain relief from compressed nerves in your spine is almost always felt in your legs, not your back.

Although stenosis and herniated discs are the two most common causes of that kind of pain, don't start thinking that a diagnosis of either one automatically makes you a candidate for a laminectomy. You know by now that back diagnoses are slippery things and that nonsurgical treatment is almost always the first, best choice. This is no exception. Although an MRI scan might show clearly that you have a herniated disc or spinal stenosis, the scan can't show whether either of these is the source of your pain. A test showing something pressing on your nerve is necessary for a laminectomy, but it is by no means sufficient.

I only recommend a laminectomy for patients who meet very specific criteria. Research has shown that patients who meet these criteria are more likely to be helped by their surgery. Patients who don't are much less likely to improve. Given how easy it is to wrongly connect pain to a finding on a test, these criteria are designed to identify patients who will benefit from having their compressed nerves relieved of pressure.

Laminectomy for a herniated disc: I have four criteria. The first one is that you have to have radicular pain. Pain that's limited to the back, or the back and buttocks, is an indication that neural impingement isn't what's causing discomfort. Second, you have to have very specific results from an imaging study. An MRI scan showing a herniated disc isn't enough; it has to show a herniated disc in the right place. For starters, it has to be at the right level. I can generally identify which nerve is causing your sciatica, and if the herniated disc is at the wrong level, there's a mismatch. (If there's a question about which nerve is involved, it may be worth getting a neurologist involved, or getting one of the tests that helps identify with greater certainty the nerve route of the sciatica, such as an EMG or a selective nerve block, which are described in chapter 6.) The disc also has to have herniated on the side that corresponds to your leg pain. If the herniation is on the right side and your pain is in your left leg, it's not the culprit.

The third criterion is that your physical exam must correspond to the nerve problem. There are many parts to the exam that can pinpoint a compressed nerve, but one part is particularly important—it's called the nerve root tension test. That sounds complicated, but it's one of the simplest tests I do. The goal is to create tension on the compressed nerve by pulling it. If your pain is down the back of your leg, I do that with a straight leg raise. You lie on a table or sit in a chair, and I raise each of your legs. If that makes pain shoot down the affected leg (and you meet the other criteria), I know that your chances of benefiting from a laminectomy are good—as high as 90 percent.[i,ii] If there's no shooting pain in the straight leg raise, your chances of success are smaller. For the much less common femoral nerve pain, which shoots down the front of the thigh, the test is similar, except that I straighten the hip (while you lie on your side) instead of lifting the leg. If that causes pain, you're a much better surgical candidate.

The fourth criterion is time. It's important that you try to wait at least six weeks to see if the symptoms improve on their own. Most people with sciatica get better within six weeks, and it's worth the wait to avoid the surgery, if you can. That is assuming that the pain was not incapacitating or that you didn't develop a neurological deficit (weakness) or signs of cauda equina syndrome (very rare, and covered in chapter 5) before the six-week mark.

There is one more issue that can affect the chance of success, although it's hard to put a number on it, and so I don't include it in my list of criteria: the size of the original herniation, particularly in relation to the size of the spinal canal. The greater the percent of the spinal canal the disc fragment takes up, the better the odds that surgery will help.[iii] So, if you have a really small disc herniation and you have a very large spinal canal, there is a lot of room for the nerves to accommodate and recover, and the chances of needing surgery are less than for someone with a larger disc and a smaller spinal canal. I wouldn't let this issue be the absolute determinant of whether you should get surgery, but if you're on the fence you might want to consider it.

If you meet these criteria, the preponderance of evidence indicates that you'll do better with a laminectomy/discectomy than without it.

SUMMARY OF CRITERIA FOR A LAMINECTOMY FOR A HERNIATED DISC

1. You have radiating pain in the leg.
2. There is a match between the location of the pain and the nerve being compressed.
3. There is a match between the herniated disc and the physical exam.
4. You've tried to wait at least six weeks.

One of the best studies of laminectomy for herniated disc was done by the Maine Lumbar Spine Study group.[iv] They followed four hundred patients, some of whom had surgery and some of whom didn't, for ten years. They found that the surgical patients did somewhat better in the leg pain department at every checkpoint: one year, five years, and ten years. Some of the patients in both the surgical and nonsurgical groups initially had back pain in addition to their leg pain, and, of those, the surgical group reported less back pain than the nonsurgical group after ten years. Don't take this as evidence that laminectomies stop back pain, though. There are other possible explanations, including the placebo effect and a kind of carryover effect from decreased leg pain. We don't fully understand how the two kinds of pain interact. All of the patients in the study had sciatica/radicular pain, which is the only kind of pain that justifies a laminectomy/discectomy.

The biggest limitation of the study was that it wasn't randomized. The patients in more severe pain were more likely to get surgery, which means the results of the two groups aren't truly comparable, but they tell us something nonetheless. Another problem was that 25 percent of the nonsurgical group went on to get surgery, and consequently had to be included in the surgical group. That could affect the scores of the nonsurgical group by removing the subjects who did so poorly without surgery that they went on to get the procedure.

There's a lot of other research about laminectomy for herniated discs, and not all of it concludes that that surgical treatment gets better results than nonsurgical treatment. A 1983 controlled, prospective study done in Norway found patients with surgical and nonsurgical treatment were faring equally well at the ten-year mark.[v] When I look at all the evidence, though, I conclude that a laminectomy works better than nonsurgical treatment for leg pain from a herniated disc.

My position on a laminectomy for a herniated disc is that if you meet all the criteria I've listed, you're more likely to have more leg pain relief by getting the surgery than by just leaving it alone. As always, the cardinal rule applies: no matter how many criteria you meet, if you can manage the pain without surgery, that is what you should do.

Laminectomy for stenosis: As with herniated discs, I have specific criteria that I think patients should meet before they consider surgery for degenerative stenosis. There are four. The first is that you have to have neurogenic claudication (pain when you walk, but not when you sit or stand or lie down; see page 48) that prevents you from walking more than a block or two. Second, neurogenic claudication has to be your primary symptom. If you're experiencing other kinds of pain, stenosis may not be the root of your problem.

The third criterion is that you have to have an imaging result that shows two things: that your stenosis is moderate to severe, and that it's central. Severity isn't a judgment call; it's a technical condition with a precise definition, and it's based on the amount of compression of the nerves in your spinal canal. If your stenosis doesn't qualify as at least moderate (and I usually only recommend surgery for severe stenosis), you may not benefit from surgery. And that "central" part is important. Most stenosis patients have central stenosis, but a few have either lateral recess stenosis or foraminal stenosis, two kinds that aren't in the middle of the spinal canal (explained on page 99). If you have either of those, and no central stenosis, there is no clear evidence that a laminectomy/decompression will effectively relieve neurogeric-claudication-related pain.[vi]

The fourth criterion is that your physical examination should be consistent with stenosis and not another condition that can mimic stenosis. We talked about vascular claudication (on page 101), but other disorders that can be picked up only by an exam need to be ruled out.

There are also factors that have nothing to do with your spinal stenosis that affect your chances of success with a laminectomy/ decompression. If you have other conditions, such as diabetes, hip arthritis, or a previous fracture of the lumbar spine, your chances of getting better with surgery are smaller.[vii]

SUMMARY OF CRITERIA FOR A LAMINECTOMY FOR SPINAL STENOSIS

1. Neurogenic claudication is the primary symptom.
2. Neurogenic claudication is severe enough to limit walking to a block or two.
3. An imaging study shows at least moderate or severe central spinal stenosis.
4. The physical exam is consistent with spinal stenosis.

The studies in the medical literature are few and most are not well done. The results, however, are consistent: surgery for stenosis seems to relieve pain well in the short and medium run, but not as well in the long run.

A 1992 review of articles on patients who had a laminectomy for spinal stenosis found an overall success rate of 64 percent.[viii] That means 64 percent of patients had an acceptable result; it does not mean that everyone had a 64 percent improvement from the surgery. The results of more recent studies are in the same ballpark.[ix] One 1996 retrospective study found that for patients with spinal stenosis who met all the criteria for surgery, the results were good at the beginning, with 85 percent of patients reporting some pain relief after the procedure. At the seven-to-ten-year follow-up, 75 percent were "satisfied," although 53 percent were unable to walk two blocks. The disconnect between subjective satisfaction (how happy they are) and objective results (how far they can walk) is one of the issues that makes analyzing data like this difficult.[x]

The Maine Lumbar Spine Study, which I talked about in the herniation section, also looked at stenosis. That study, published in 2005, followed surgical and nonsurgical patients with spinal stenosis. Leg pain relief and functional status improved more in the surgery group than in the nonsurgery group. After eight to ten years, 66.7 percent of the subjects who'd had surgery reported reduced leg pain, compared to 40.5 percent of the subjects who hadn't had surgery. Back pain and overall satisfaction, however, were similar in the two groups.[xi]

Some of those numbers may look pretty promising to you, especially if you're in pain and other treatments haven't worked. You can't make the decision about surgery without comparing it to other possibilities. In the case of stenosis, we don't have great comparisons, but we can take a stab at it. A study done at the Hospital for Special Surgery in New York looked at patients with central stenosis. Among those with radicular pain, half saw an improvement in their pain after three years with what the authors called "aggressive nonsurgical treatment," which included physical therapy, analgesics, and epidural injections.[xii] Their conclusion was that nonoperative treatment for lumbar stenosis remains a reasonable alternative to surgical intervention.

If you meet the criteria I outlined, you may be a candidate for a laminectomy. It's hard to say for sure, though, because although laminectomy is the most commonly performed back operation in the United States, and stenosis is one of the top two reasons patients get a laminectomy, I have not been able to unearth one single piece of prospective, randomized, controlled research on a laminectomy versus nonoperative treatment for leg pain caused by stenosis.

In 2006, the American Academy of Orthopaedic Surgeons published *OKU: Orthopaedic Knowledge Update Spine 3*, a reference for orthopedic surgeons, residents, and students. Their frustration on this topic was palpable:

A recent review of the literature did not identify a randomized controlled trial comparing surgical versus nonsurgical treatment. An attempted meta-analysis of the literature on surgical outcomes for patients with lumbar spinal stenosis concluded that the poor scientific quality of the literature precluded conducting the intended meta-analysis.[xiii]

The good news is that you don't have to choose, at least not today. If you're considering surgery, there's no harm in putting it off while you try other treatments. Nothing terrible will happen if you decide to postpone. You're not going to wake up paralyzed. You can always have the surgery next year. Who knows, in that year your pain may subside to the point where you can live without surgery.

My recommendation is that you consider the criteria I've outlined very carefully. If you meet them, surgery is a good option.

CASE STUDY

JEFF is a retired teacher in his seventies. He came to see me with an MRI that showed very severe spinal stenosis. He'd been told he needed surgery, but he was planning a trip to Italy. When I asked him about walking, he told me he could walk a mile easily and had no leg pain. He wasn't worried that his mild back pain would limit him on the trip—but that he'd miss the trip altogether while he was recuperating from surgery. This was a man who was fully functional. And while the stenosis was clear on his MRI, Jeff simply didn't need surgery. It's likely that he may show up in my office with leg pain one of these days, but he hasn't yet (he keeps in touch with me), and I wouldn't dream of recommending surgery until he does.

LAMINECTOMY FOR OTHER DIAGNOSES

Although herniated discs and spinal stenosis are the two most common reasons to get a lumbar laminectomy, there are many others. The list is long and varied: shattered bones, spinal nerve tumors, cysts, infections, abscesses, and hematomas. What they have in common (besides rarity) is that they all require access to the spinal canal.

Many of these are emergencies and urgencies; those things have to be removed when they're pushing on your nerves, and a laminectomy is the easiest way we have to do that. There is one special case that I do want to mention, though. If you have a vertebral compression fracture, a laminectomy is generally a bad idea. Once the vertebra collapses, the job of keeping your spine stable falls to the lamina and the facet joints. If you take out a piece of the lamina, you really do risk instability. A laminectomy is almost never needed in that situation, but if it is, a fusion is also usually called for.

LAMINECTOMY SUMMARY
- Laminectomy/discectomy relieves the shooting leg pain that comes from a herniated disc.
- Laminectomy/decompression relieves the pain you have when walking that comes from spinal stenosis.
- In either case, make sure you meet the specific criteria to maximize the chance of benefiting from the procedure.

WHEN NOT TO GET A LAMINECTOMY

In short, laminectomies aren't good for back pain. Laminectomies are effective for nerve-related leg pain. While a laminectomy can fix pain that emanates from a compressed nerve, it won't fix your problem if a compressed nerve isn't the cause.

I have known surgeons to recommend a laminectomy for back pain—that is, surgeons who are flat-out wrong—but it doesn't happen that often. In my experience, the misapplication of the procedure is more subtle. When a patient has both back pain and leg pain, and some kind of stenosis or herniation, it's easy to jump to the laminectomy conclusion. But if you don't meet the specific criteria I outlined above, your chances of success are mediocre at best.

Another common misuse of a laminectomy is for the wrong kind of stenosis. Only central stenosis, not lateral recess or foraminal stenosis, is likely to cause the nerve compression symptoms (neurogenic claudication) that a laminectomy/decompression will relieve. Most of my patients figure that stenosis is stenosis is stenosis, and don't ever dig any deeper; they have stenosis, and they know that laminectomies get done for stenosis, end of story. But the details matter. If you're considering a laminectomy, make sure you meet all the criteria I outlined above. If you're not sure, talk to your doctor.

The same holds true for herniated discs. Some patients come to see me knowing only that they've been diagnosed with one, but they don't know which side it's on or how severe it is. If the disc has herniated on the right, but the nerve-related pain is on the left, a laminectomy/discectomy is not going to relieve your pain.

Unfortunately, there is no magic test strip that turns green if you need a laminectomy and purple if you don't. We can't always tell beyond a shadow of a doubt that whatever is compressing your nerve(s) is indeed the source of the pain. Even meeting very specific criteria, developed from a comprehensive review of the evidence, isn't a guarantee that surgery will work. It can, however, dramatically increase your chances that a laminectomy will be a success, and reduce your chances of having the surgery inappropriately.

WHAT CAN GO WRONG

A laminectomy is a relatively straightforward procedure with few serious complications. The one important risk you need to be aware of is spondylolisthesis, an out-of-line vertebra. If your doctor removes too much bone from the facet joint or the pars interarticularis, both of which are right next door to the lamina, the vertebra can no longer hold its place in line with your spine, and it slips out of place. As I pointed out in chapter 1, there is no official border between the lamina and the pars interarticularis. I have known cases in which a surgeon has felt the need to remove some of the lamina, and then a little more, and then a little more, until enough of the facet joint or pars interarticularis was gone to cause instability. It doesn't happen often, but it does happen. The problem might or might not require revision surgery; it depends on how significant the slippage is and how much pain the problem causes.

I want to emphasize that simply removing the lamina doesn't cause instability. If it did, a laminectomy wouldn't be the safe procedure it is. Your vertebrae are thick, strong bones, and you can remove the entire lamina from several of them without jeopardizing your spine's ability to hold you up.

There is also a chance that your doctor will make a mistake. He's maneuvering in a tight space, and it is possible, but rare, that he will cut a nerve or cause a leak of spinal fluid. It is also possible, but rare, that your surgeon could operate at the wrong site. Two preventable reasons laminectomies go wrong are that doctors operate on the wrong vertebra or on the wrong side of the correct vertebra. Nobody collects statistics on this, so I can't tell you how often it happens. My prediction, though, is that it will happen less and less often. In the last few years there's been a national initiative on wrong site surgery, and doctors and hospitals are incorporating simple preventive measures into their standard operating procedures.

To make sure that the above doesn't happen to you, talk to your surgeon and to the nurse who preps you for surgery. Make sure that everyone understands precisely what surgery you're getting, including which level and which side it's on (for a herniated disc). You can even ask your surgeon to write it on your back, while you are awake, in indelible ink, just to make sure. This way, when they turn you over, it's right there in front of the doctor.

The risk of paralysis, which is the risk I find my patients are most worried about, is very, very small.

All that said, the vast majority of laminectomies come off without a hitch, with patients unable to tell that anything's changed. Your laminae are too deeply buried in your body to feel them from the surface, and the only evidence a successful laminectomy will leave behind is no more pain and a small scar.

LAMINECTOMY AND FUSION

One of the misuses of a laminectomy has nothing to do with the laminectomy itself. It's the increasing prevalence of doing a spinal fusion along with it. I think there are two reasons the practice of doing the two procedures together is on the rise. The first is that the rationale for adding fusion to a laminectomy is based on instability, a very malleable concept. The second is that patients, once they've decided to get a laminectomy, figure that adding a fusion is no big deal.

I want to tackle the instability issue first. Laminectomy candidates have a clear-cut diagnosis based on an abnormality that shows up on a test, usually compression of a nerve by a herniated disc or constriction (stenosis) of the spinal canal. The laminectomy is performed specifically to relieve pressure on a nerve that the abnormality is causing, but it's easy to speculate that the same abnormality may also be causing "instability" that is contributing to your back pain, and therefore that a fusion is necessary. That is rarely the case.

Here's where we run into trouble. Pressure on a nerve and "instability" can coexist, but they don't necessarily. Pressure on a nerve is an objective finding, but "instability" is a condition with a vague definition and lot of wiggle room. Nevertheless, it's what most doctors base their fusion recommendation on.

There are criteria for instability, which I describe in the fusion chapter on page 208, and if your doctor tells you your spine is "unstable," you should ask him to be more specific. Is your spine unstable as it is, or do you have a condition that could become unstable after the laminectomy? Determining whether you have one of these conditions usually requires an

X-ray to look for a structural problem, such as spondylolisthe-sis or scoliosis, or flexion and extension X-rays to find abnor-mal motion between two vertebrae over the threshold defined as "stable."

Alternatively, your doctor might recommend fusion if you have a lot of back pain (along with the leg pain for which you're getting a laminectomy), even if you don't have genuine instability to start with or a condition that might result in instability after the laminectomy. If he does, you need to know that there is no solid evidence that a fusion will relieve your back pain.[xiv,xv] Re-gardless of what prompts your surgeon's recommendation of fu-sion to go with your laminectomy, be sure to read the chapter on spinal fusion.

Which brings me to the second factor. Once you've made a de-cision to have surgery, you've crossed a mental threshold. You've carefully weighed the risks and benefits that come with that. The idea of doing a fusion while your surgeon is already in there doesn't seem like such a big deal; after all, you're getting surgery anyhow. But it *is* a big deal. Fusion is a much riskier procedure than a laminectomy. You have to consider a fusion done in con-junction with a laminectomy just as carefully as you consider a stand-alone spinal fusion. Don't ever do it as an afterthought or an insurance policy.

Laminectomy and fusion: two procedures, two decisions. Con-sider the decision to add fusion to your laminectomy just as carefully as you'd consider a stand-alone fusion. The fusion-laminectomy combination is much riskier than a laminectomy alone.

WHEN YOU SHOULD CONSIDER FUSION WITH A LAMINECTOMY

There are some genuinely destabilizing conditions that should make you consider the possibility of a fusion in conjunction with your laminectomy. If you have spondylolisthesis, you have the potential to be unstable. The same is true if you have scoliosis. If you have lateral listhesis, a sideways slippage of the bones, you should strongly consider a fusion. If a disc reherniates more than twice (that is, you're going in for your third laminectomy on the same disc), you should also consider fusion, because, in theory at least, preventing motion will also prevent yet another recurrence of the herniation.

Whatever your diagnosis, be sure you make the fusion decision independent of the laminectomy. It's not like picking up the dry cleaning because you're already out for the groceries.

CASE STUDY

PATRICK is a fireman in his mid-fifties who's been injured several times on the job in spectacular ways, such as falling through roofs. He came to me with symptoms of spinal stenosis. I ran tests and found that he had also a stable grade I spondylolisthesis (about 10 percent at the same level as the stenosis). He could barely walk—he had crippling neurologic claudication. But he had no back pain. The two problems needed to be considered together yet separately. The stenosis was causing his pain. He had no pain from his spondylolisthesis, and flexion and extension X-rays showed no movement of the bones at all. Patrick was a runner, and he wanted desperately to get back to running. We talked about his two separate but related problems, and decided that for him and his goals the best plan was to do a laminectomy for the stenosis, but leave the spondylolisthesis alone. We both knew we'd have to watch the spondylolisthesis closely. Two years later, Patrick is pain-free, his spondylolisthesis remains at 10 percent, and he is back running!

SUCCESS RATES FOR THE FUSION-LAMINECTOMY COMBINATION

If you're considering the combo for a herniated disc, and are looking for hard data to help you make a hard decision, you're out of luck. There is, as yet, no data on pain outcomes for laminectomies with and without fusion for herniated discs. Until we have it, and it shows compellingly that the outcomes are better for both procedures (don't hold your breath), take your surgery one step at a time.

For spinal stenosis we do have some data. The statistic that may be scariest is how often the two surgeries are being done together. From 1996 to 2001 (the last year for which we have analyzed data), the rate of fusion being done for degenerative conditions in the United States *doubled*. Indeed, by 2001 over half of all inpatient lumbar spine surgery, other than that for herniated discs, included a fusion procedure. Fusion rates associated with herniated discs also rose sharply.[xvi]

But does it work? There are many studies that find that a laminectomy with fusion relieves back pain (although not leg pain) better than a laminectomy alone. Unfortunately, most of them were not controlled, randomized, or prospective. And they lumped patients with lots of different conditions together. When some subjects have back pain, some have scoliosis, and some have spondylolisthesis, it's hard to tease out the results for the patients with a specific condition or instability.

One of the first prospective (but not randomized or controlled) studies was done in 1997, and it compared three groups, all of whom had neurogenic claudication (leg pain with walking) from stenosis. One group had a laminectomy, one group had a laminectomy with fusion, and the third group had a laminectomy with fusion done with implants. Interestingly, the main determinant of who got a laminectomy and who got a laminectomy with fusion was not the underlying condition, but the surgeon's preference. At the six-month and twenty-four-month checkpoints, the laminectomy with noninstrumented fusion outperformed both the laminectomy alone and the instrumented fusion for back pain, although not by much.[xvii] While this study is compelling, other studies have found no difference in the pain relief from a laminectomy and a laminectomy with fusion.[xviii]

It's also worth noting that, with fusion, the complication rates go way up (more on that in chapter 13). A study done in 1993 on Medicare patients found that the risk of complications doubled when fusion was added into the mix.[xix]

Here's my recommendation. If you have stenosis or a herniated disc that is severe enough to be treated with a laminectomy, there are a few conditions for which you should consider fusion. If you have spondylolisthesis, scoliosis, or both, or if your surgeon is going to have to remove a significant amount of facet or pars interarticularis bone, along with the lamina, you are at risk for instability. If you don't, there's no reason to think that a fusion will relieve your back pain (and remember, the laminectomy is for your leg pain).

The odds change if the surgery you're having is revision surgery. The second or third time around, the odds that a laminectomy will indeed put you at risk for instability are higher, and you might consider a fusion. I talk about this more in chapter 18: Revision Surgery.

RECOVERY

For a laminectomy because of a herniated disc, about half my patients leave the hospital the same day, and half leave the next morning, usually depending on their preference. For stenosis, most patients spend two to four days in the hospital. The recovery takes longer because stenosis surgery generally involves more bone removal, and the patients are usually older. The incisions are bigger and the muscle dissection (moving the muscle off the bone) is more substantial, because it has to be done on both sides. The surgery takes longer, you're under anesthesia longer, and the recovery is commensurately longer.

Once you're up and out of bed, though, my recommendations are the same no matter which kind of laminectomy you had (as long as it didn't include fusion). If you're having trouble getting out of bed, or with walking, a physical therapist can help you get back on your feet, and strong enough to leave the hospital. For the first six weeks, you should avoid bending, twisting, and lifting—but you should walk. Walk a lot. It's the best thing you can do to get your body functioning normally again. The worst thing you can do is lie in bed.

You may not get these identical instructions from your doctor. Every doctor is different, and since there isn't a lot of data, we each rely on our own experience.

ENDNOTES

i L. F. Supik, M. J. Broom, "Sciatic Tension Signs and Lumbar Disc Hernia-tion," *Spine* 19, no. 9 (1994), pp. 1066–69.

ii Xin Shiqing, Zhang Quanzhi, and Fan Dehao, "Significance of the Straight-Leg-Raising Test in the Diagnosis and Clinical Evaluation of Lower Lumbar Intervertebral-Disc Protrusion," *Journal of Bone and Joint Surgery (Am.)* 69 (1987), pp. 517–22.

iii E. J. Carragee, D. H. Kim, "A Prospective Analysis of Magnetic Resonance Imaging Findings in Patients With Sciatica and Lumbar Disc Herniation: Correlation of Outcomes with Disc Fragment and Canal Morphology," *Spine* 22, no. 14 (1997), pp. 1650–60.

iv S. J. Atlas, et al., "Long-term Outcomes of Surgical and Nonsurgical Man-agement of Sciatica Secondary to a Lumbar Disc Herniation: 10 year Re-sults from the Maine Lumbar Spine Study," *Spine* 30, no. 8 (2005), pp. 927–35.

v H. Weber, "Lumbar Disc Herniation: A Controlled, Prospective Study with Ten Years of Observation," *Spine* 8, no. 2 (1983), pp. 131–40.

vi J.N.A. Gibson, G. Waddell, "Surgery for Degenerative Lumbar Spondylo-sis: Updated Cochrane Review," *Spine* 30 (2005), pp. 2312–20.

vii O. Airaksinen, et al., "Surgical Outcome of 438 Patients Treated Surgi-cally for Lumbar Spinal Stenosis," *Spine* 22 (1997), pp. 2278–82.

viii J. A. Turner, M. Ersek, L. Herron, et al., "Surgery for Lumbar Spinal Steno-sis: Attempted Meta-analysis of the Literature," *Spine* 17, no. 1 (1992), pp. 1–8.

ix T. Iguchi, et al. "Minimum 10-year Outcome of Decompressive Laminec-tomy for Degenerative Lumbar Spinal Stenosis," *Spine* 25, no. 14 (2000), pp. 1754–59.

x J. Katz, et al., Seven- to 10-year Outcome of Decompressive Surgery for Degenerative Lumbar Spinal Stenosis, *Spine* 21, no. 1 (1996), pp. 92–97.

xi S. J. Atlas, et al., "Long-term Outcomes of Surgical and Nonsurgical Man-agement of Lumbar Spinal Stenosis: 8 to 10 Year Results from the Maine Lumbar Spine Study," *Spine* 30, no. 8 (2005), pp. 936–43.

xii A. C. Simotas, et al., "Nonoperative Treatment for Lumbar Spinal Steno-sis: Clinical and Outcome Results and a 3-year Survivorship Analysis," *Spine* 25, no. 2 (2000), pp. 197–204.

xiii American Academy of Orthopaedic Surgeons, *OKU: Orthopaedic Knowledge Update: Spine* 3 (2006), p. 303.

xiv D. K. Resnick, T. F. Choudhri, A. T. Dailey, et al., "Guidelines for the Performance of Fusion Procedures for Degenerative Disease of the Lumbar Spine. Part 8: Lumbar Fusion for Disc Herniation and Radiculopathy," *Journal of Neurosurgery Spine* 2 (2005), pp. 673–78.

xv Ibid., "Part 10: Fusion Following Decompression in Patients with Stenosis Without Spondylolisthesis," pp. 686–91.

xvi R. A. Deyo, et al., "United States Trends in Lumbar Fusion Surgery for Degenerative Conditions," *Spine* 30, no. 12 (2005), pp. 1441–45.

xvii J. N. Katz, et al., "Lumbar Laminectomy Alone or with Instrumented or Noninstrumented Arthrodesis in Degenerative Lumbar Spinal Stenosis: Patient Selection, Costs, and Surgical Outcomes," *Spine* 22, no. 10 (1997), pp. 1123–31.

xviii D. Grob, T. Humke, J. Dvorak, "Degenerative Lumbar Spinal Stenosis. Decompression With and Without Arthrodesis," *Journal of Bone and Joint Surgery (Am.)* 77, no. 7 (1995), pp. 1036–41.

xix R. A. Deyo, et al., "Lumbar Spinal Fusion. A Cohort Study of Complications, Reoperations, and Resource Use in the Medicare Population," *Spine* 18, no. 11 (1993), pp. 1463–70.

Chapter 13

SPINAL FUSION

One of the reasons things go wrong so often in the spine is that it has a lot of moving parts. One way to stop pain is to immobilize the parts causing the pain. That's what spinal fusion does. If one particular disc or one unstable vertebra is the source of your pain, then fusing the bones on either side of the problem should relieve it.

To understand what fusion does, think of your spine as a train. The vertebrae are the cars, and the discs and facet joints allow for movement—they're the couplings. Since the cars themselves don't bend, but the train needs to go around curves, the couplings between the cars have to allow for motion but also be strong enough to keep the cars together. It's the same with your spine. Fusion takes two (or sometimes more) of the vertebrae, eliminates the flexible coupling in between, and binds the vertebrae together to yield one inflexible unit.

The decision to get fusion surgery—also called arthrodesis—is one of the most difficult my patients face. To make it, you have to understand what fusion can and can't do, what the differences are among the varieties of fusion, and which varieties best treat which conditions. On top of that, you have to understand the basics of bone grafts (which I explain at the end of this chapter) and implants (which have a chapter all their own). If you're facing the decision, that may sound like a daunting list, but I assure you that by the end of this chapter you'll know just about everything you need to know. Granted, it's a long chapter, but a lot hangs in the balance.

Ready? Take a deep breath, and let's start with the first, and fundamental, question of what fusion's good for.

WHY FUSION?

To understand what fusion can successfully treat, you have to answer one important question: is your pain related to instability? If it is, the theory behind fusion is easy to understand. Fusion takes all motion out of the equation by fusing the problem area into one immobile unit. Without motion, there can be no instability in the fused part of the spine. No instability, no pain—hopefully.

If your pain isn't related to instability, and is thought to be coming from a disc, the theory is a little different. Some people speculate that a disc can be painful in and of itself. If the disc is painful because there's something "wrong" with it (and "wrong" can mean any of the discogenic pain diagnoses—degenerated disc, black disc, IDD), then the pain may have nothing to do with motion. It is the disc itself that hurts, and if we remove it and fuse the two vertebrae around it, we take the problem disc out of commission and thereby stop the pain.

Although these two explanations are equally simple, they are not equally well accepted. Fusion's ability to solve problems stemming from instability-related pain is well documented. Fusion's ability to stop pain that's not related to instability is highly suspect.

Unfortunately, there is a trend in the United States toward doing more fusions for the latter. Fusion originated at the turn of the twentieth century to treat instability-generating conditions, such as severe scoliosis, fractures, and spinal tuberculosis. In those cases, fusion continues to be a lifesaving treatment. In the case of a burst fracture where the spinal cord is in danger, fusion is indispensable. For scoliosis, fusion can straighten and stabilize the spine. Whenever there's a true mechanical dissociation of the bones, fusion is the only option.

In the five years from 1996 to 2001, however, the number of fusions performed in this country for nontraumatic conditions increased by 113 percent.[i] There are now estimated to be at least 200,000 fusions done every year,[ii] and all indications are that the number is going nowhere but up. It's a pretty safe bet that more people aren't getting scoliosis, fractures, and tuberculosis. What's driving the increase is the gradual acceptance of fusion as a treatment for back pain. Today three-quarters of spinal fusions are done to treat disc disorders, spinal degeneration, and stenosis.[iii]

It's this trend that makes it so important that you understand when fusion is appropriate and when it isn't. Let's start with when it is.

FUSION FOR INSTABILITY-RELATED PAIN

As I mentioned in the previous chapter, the definition of spinal instability is muddy enough to leave a lot of wiggle room, and it's probably one of the most abused terms in the spine field. At the risk of overwhelming you with med-speak, I want to give you verbatim examples of the definition of the two kinds of instability doctors talk about: clinical and radiologic.

Clinical: Loss of the ability of the spine under physiologic loads to maintain its pattern of displacement so that there is no initial or additional neurologic deficit, no major deformity, and no incapacitating pain.[iv]

Radiologic: The amount of sagittal rotation observed between the extremes of movement (on flexion-extension radiographs) or the amount of vertebral rotation. Typically, values of 10 degrees for rotation and 4 millimeters for translation are used to infer instability.[v]

Now that I've done my due diligence by giving you the letter of the law, I'll explain it in plain English. Clinical instability is when you have abnormal motion between two spinal segments that results in severe deformity or pain or neurological compromise when you do ordinary things, such as walking, sitting, or standing. Radiologic instability is defined by the results of flexion and extension X-rays (described on page 78), which can show abnormal motion by comparing the unstable segment to its neighbors. If the vertebra in that segment slides more than four millimeters over the adjacent one, or the difference between the flexion and extension angles is more than ten degrees, that's instability.

It seems, from the clinical definition, that it would be easy to tell if your spine is unstable. And certainly you'd think you'd know if you have a severe deformity or pain or neurological compromise. But both definitions, and particularly the radiological, are such that you could have what a doctor would call instability and still feel perfectly fine. Despite many attempts to refine these definitions, what often isn't said in discussions of instability is that it frequently doesn't cause pain. One review article of research on fusion for chronic pain put it succinctly: "Although many surgeons rely on these [clinical and radiologic] guidelines, there is no data that clearly links pain with instability."[vi]

This brings us full circle to one of the recurring themes of this book: the difficulty of pegging pain to a specific source. If you've got what your doctor describes as instability, and you've also got pain, there is no guarantee that the instability causes the pain.

Much of this book is dedicated to convincing you to worry less about treating your diagnosis and more about treating your pain. If you're considering fusion, though, the key consideration is the underlying diagnosis. The only way to know whether your pain is likely to respond to fusion is to know that it's coming from instability, and the way to establish that it's coming from instability is to find a definitive cause of that instability. If your doctor finds radiological instability, there's a big difference between attributing it to a degenerated disc, which we're not certain can cause instability, and attributing it to spondylolisthesis, which can absolutely cause instability.

There are several potentially destabilizing conditions we understand quite well, and for which fusion is a well-accepted treatment.

Spondylolisthesis is a condition in which a vertebra slips out of the lineup. It has a number of causes, but in adults it is most likely related to facet arthritis or spondylolysis, a fracture of the pars interarticularis. If either spondylolisthesis or spondylolysis is severe it can cause both instability and pain. In both cases, surgery has a good record of alleviating pain.

Tumors and infections can invade bones and make them weak. If they weaken to the point of breaking or your surgeon needs to resect enough of the tumor to destabilize the spine, the result can be serious pain and possible irreparable neurological damage. Fusing the bones above and below the weakened bone can prevent that.

Fractures cause instability for obvious reasons. If the bone is broken, it can't do its job. Fusion can take the place of a bone that can't support your body without pain, nerve damage, or further collapsing.

Scoliosis and kyphosis are curvatures of the spine that can range from minor to severe (scoliosis is lateral, kyphosis is front-to-back). Large curves can cause pain and make even standing or walking difficult. Fusion can realign the spine to a better position, and stabilize it so it doesn't curve any further.

Revision surgery is a broad category, and encompasses everything from pseudarthrosis to recurrent herniated disc.

Fusion has a good track record treating severe cases of all of these conditions, which are explained in more detail in their respective chapters. (Spondylolysis, spondylolisthesis, scoliosis, and kyphosis are covered in chapter 7; fractures, tumors, and infections are covered in chapter 5. I cover revision surgery in chapter 18.)

If you're considering surgery for any of these, remember my mantra: if your pain is manageable and your condition doesn't threaten vital structures, it's best to avoid surgery.

FUSION FOR BACK PAIN WITHOUT INSTABILITY

This is one of the most important sections of the book. It's the single biggest reason I decided to write it. If it's even crossed your mind to get fusion surgery for back pain, I want you to read it very carefully. I'll warn you ahead of time that there's a lot of data in this section. I would have spared you some of it if I'd thought that I could give you a fair assessment of fusion for back pain without it. But that's not possible, so you're going to have to bear with me.

Although there is a lot of research on the topic, there isn't a consensus. The rate of success of fusion for low back pain is anywhere from 16 percent to 95 percent, depending on who you ask.[vii] One reason is that most of the research is not first-rate. There are, however, three randomized, controlled studies, all done in the last several years, that compare fusion with various kinds of nonoperative treatment. These studies are the best information we have, and they're the basis of my recommendations.

The first is a study done in Sweden. It garnered a lot of attention, won an award, and is often cited in support of performing fusion for back pain. It found that patients who got fusion did better after two years than patients who didn't. The study followed 294 very carefully selected participants who were randomly assigned to fusion surgery or something other than surgery (the treatment was left to the doctors' discretion, and ranged from acupuncture to physical therapy). After two years, the group that got the surgery had, on average, a third less pain than before, compared to a measly 7 percent decrease in the nonsurgical group.[viii] On the face of it, that's a pretty strong argument that getting fusion surgery is better than other things if you've got back pain.

It's a conclusion that should be interpreted cautiously, however, and one of the reasons is that the Swedish study, like most studies, has some important limitations. Its two biggest problems are its short duration and the type of treatment the nonsurgical group got. The short duration is a problem because fusion surgery for back pain should, in theory, be a lifelong solution. You're taking the disc permanently out of play, and so it shouldn't give you any more trouble (although other discs might). Two years isn't nearly long enough to assess what is supposed to be a long-term treatment, particularly since the surgical group experienced the greatest pain relief in the first six months after surgery, when you would expect any placebo effect to be strongest. After those six months, the group's pain started to increase, and continued its steady climb up for the eighteen months remaining in the study. If that trend continued after the two-year mark, those patients would end up pretty close to where they began, or maybe worse. We don't know how they fared in the long term. (Apparently, the authors of the study did some longer-term follow-up, but they have yet to publish those results.)

The second problem, common to many studies that compare surgical and nonsurgical treatments, is that the group who didn't get surgery got a variety of treatments, none of which were described. Some of them may have been effective and some of them may not have been. Ideally, we'd like to see surgery compared with the most effective nonsurgical treatment. That's the choice any rational patient wants to make.

The other two studies don't support the conclusions of the Swedish study. In fact, they both found very little difference in outcomes between surgery and specific nonoperative treatments. The first, published in 2003, followed sixty-four patients for a year. They were randomly assigned to get either fusion surgery or treatment that consisted of cognitive intervention and a three-week exercise program. After a year, the surgery group had slightly more improvement in pain and disability scores, but they also had an 18 percent complication rate. The authors concluded: "The main outcome measure showed equal improvement" in both groups.[ix] The second study, this one from 2005, had 349 participants assigned to either fusion surgery or an intensive rehabilitation program. The study also found slightly more improvement, on some scores, in the fusion group, but not enough to justify the risk or the cost. "No clear evidence emerged that primary spinal fusion surgery was any more beneficial than intensive rehabilitation."[x]

If you read the early chapters of this book, this is a conclusion that shouldn't surprise you. You already know that it's hard to figure out where pain comes from. It's hard to decide if it's coming from a disc, let alone which disc it's coming from. It's possible that discs don't even cause pain. With all that uncertainty, low success rates are almost inevitable.

Nevertheless, I've included the best research we have in some detail because the conclusion that I draw from them, and the conclusion that I think you should draw from them, runs contrary to the recommendation that many doctors make. It seems clear to me that the fairly small benefits of fusion surgery for low back pain don't outweigh the risks, though obviously other doctors disagree or there wouldn't be 200,000 patients getting spinal fusion every year.

> **Spinal fusion for back pain with instability is not the same as spinal fusion for back pain without instability.** If you meet the criteria for instability and you have pain, surgery may work wonders. If you only have pain, and no instability, surgical results are not nearly as predictable.

There have been several attempts by spine doctors to make sense of all this research and decide once and for all whether fusion can help with low back pain. One such attempt, the results of which were published in 2005, concluded that, when it came to degenerative back pain, "there is still insufficient evidence on the effectiveness of surgery on clinical outcomes to draw any firm conclusions."[xi] Another review, published in 2004, gave a hint to its conclusion in its title: "Spinal-Fusion Surgery—The Case for Restraint." According to that article, which expressed skepticism about fusion's effectiveness for many conditions and alarm at its growing prevalence, "there are conflicting results from clinical trials and small benefits at best from spinal fusion among patients with diskogenic pain," and that "more evidence from clinical trials should be required for degenerative disk disease to be an accepted indication [for fusion]."[xii]

Not everyone agrees with these assessments. There's a raging controversy in the spine community about what fusion can and can't do. There are many surgeons who believe that, for a carefully selected group of patients, fusion can alleviate discogenic low back pain. Generally, they hang their collective hat on the Swedish study that showed fusion to best advantage.

That controversy has remained primarily confined to spinal doctors. Very little of the back-and-forth on the issue has made it to the mainstream press, and patients haven't been part of the discussion. If the debate had been playing out in the pages of *Newsweek* rather than the medical journal *Spine*, I suspect patients would have started balking at fusion for back pain long ago.

For me, the controversy isn't very controversial. I think the evidence so far is clear. After looking exhaustively at the research (the studies I've cited, as well as many that I haven't), I have to conclude that, if you have back pain, your chance of getting better with fusion is about the same as your chance of getting better with an effective, nonoperative treatment program. That, in a nutshell, is the most important fact in this book. It's the fact I opened with, it's the fact that is fueling a fight in the medical community, and it's the fact that's most likely to do the largest number of back patients some good.

THE VARIETIES OF FUSION

By the time you get to this point in the chapter, you should have a good idea whether your particular condition makes you a candidate for fusion surgery. If it does, you need to understand the procedure itself. Fusion comes in many forms, from a relatively straightforward one-level, noninstrumented, posterolateral procedure to a multilevel, instrumented, circumferential procedure. I do

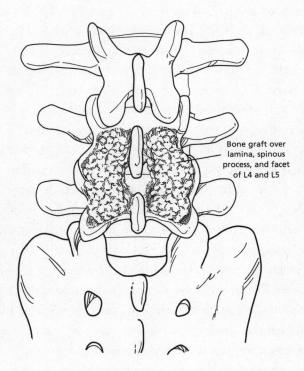

Bone graft over lamina, spinous process, and facet of L4 and L5

In a posterior fusion, the spinous processes, laminae and facets are fused as shown above. If possible, the transverse processes are also fused (not shown).

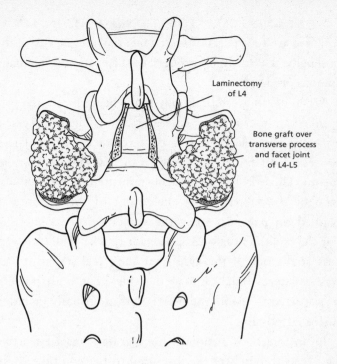

Laminectomy
of L4

Bone graft over
transverse process
and facet joint
of L4-L5

In a posterolateral fusion, the facets and transverse processes are
fused to their neighbors. Note the missing lamina and spinous
process.

a lot of both kinds; I might do the simplest kind for a spondylolisthesis patient one day, and the most complex kind for a multiple
trauma victim the next. I see firsthand not only the differences in
complexity but also the differences in risk and recovery time.

If you're thinking about fusion, you also need to understand
those differences. The three fundamental considerations in fusion
surgery are what to fuse, how to get access to it, and whether to
use instrumentation.

WHAT GETS FUSED: LOCATION, LOCATION, LOCATION

There are four parts of your spine that can be fused: the vertebral body, the transverse process, the facet and the lamina (with its spinous process).

When it's the vertebral body that's being fused, the procedure is called an interbody, or anterior, fusion. The transverse process is fused to its neighbor in a posterolateral fusion. The spinous process and laminae are fused to their neighbors in a posterior fusion. Those last two are easily confused, but you'll keep them straight if you remember the layout of the vertebra (it's explained on page 5). Since the spinous process sticks straight out the back, its fusion is posterior (back). The transverse process sticks out of the side (you can't feel it), so its fusion is posterolateral (back and to the side). For both posterior and posterolateral fusion, the facet joints are usually included in the fusion, if possible.

In an interbody fusion, a bone graft is inserted between the two vertebrae, where the disc used to be (you take it out to do the procedure). It holds the vertebrae together like peanut butter between two slices of bread. For posterior and posterolateral fusion, the bone graft is placed next to the vertebrae, and the graft holds the bones together like the spine of a comb holds the teeth.

There are circumstances when it is particularly important that a fusion fuses solid; they don't always, as you'll find out as you continue reading. In that case, your surgeon may opt for the belt-and-suspenders approach of combined fusion, which combines an interbody with a posterior fusion so you get the peanut butter *and* the comb spine. (You may also see combined fusion called circumferential fusion, front-back fusion, or 360-degree fusion.)

No matter the type of fusion, the procedure is the same in

principle. The surgeon scrapes away the surface of whatever's going to be fused to reveal a raw surface of bone at the site where the bone graft is going to go. This is essentially a trick to get your bones to fuse to the bone graft. When bone is scraped down, it tries to heal itself by forming new bone. If the inserted bone is there when that happens, the bone will often (but not always) graft itself onto it. Voilà! Fusion!

FRONT OR BACK: THE ACCESS POINT

Some fusions are done through your back, and others through your front. Posterior and posterolateral fusion can only be done through the back. Interbody fusions can be done either through your back or through your front, and each method has its advantages and disadvantages. There are lots of reasons to choose one access point or the other, but the most basic is which part of your spine is causing trouble. If it's the disc (not a herniated disc, but a disc suspected of causing pain), it makes sense to go in through the front, where you get the best access to it. If it's a broken facet, it makes sense to go in through the back for the same reason.

If you're getting an interbody fusion that's done through the back, you need to know the specifics. There are two ways to do the surgery. A posterior lumbar interbody fusion (PLIF) goes directly through the back of the spine, and requires that the spinous process and laminae be removed and the nerves pushed out of the way to get access to the disc. A transforaminal lumbar interbody fusion (TLIF) goes through the back but off to the side of the spine, and requires that the facet joint be removed to get access to the disc.

One problem with PLIF is that the nerves must be moved aside to get access to the disc space. This is why the odds of nerve

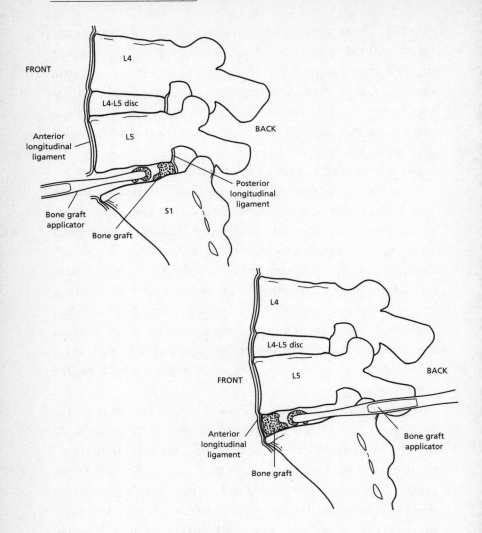

Anterior lumbar interbody fusion is done from the front, as shown on the upper left; posterior lumbar interbody fusions (PLIF or TLIF) are done from the back, as shown on the lower right.

damage are higher with PLIF than they are with TLIF. The problem with TLIF is that removing the facet joint destabilizes the spine, and so TLIFs almost always have to be instrumented (PLIFs are almost always instrumented as well, but the danger of destabilization is smaller). It's impossible to say that one is, all things considered, safer than the other, and the kind you should get is probably the kind your surgeon prefers. I prefer TLIFs, but I know fine surgeons who prefer PLIFs.

If you're following this, you may be wondering why, if a surgeon is going to remove the disc, he doesn't just go in from the front and take it out. That procedure also has a name, anterior lumbar interbody fusion (ALIF), and it's often used to remove a problem disc. But if your problem involves a herniated disc or stenosis, or anything else that is inside the spinal canal, it's almost impossible to remove it from the front. Your surgeon doesn't have the view or the access or the accuracy to work through the depth of the vertebral body, starting at the front, to reach the back. It's too dangerous.

Anterior fusions, which are only interbody, can be done in one of two ways. The ALIF is done directly through your front, and its close cousin the XLIF (extreme lateral lumbar interbody fusion; the second L gets dropped in the acronym) is done at a slightly different angle, through your flank. XLIF is only a couple of years old, so it is too early to say whether it's better or safer.

ALIFs and XLIFs are for stabilizing the spine when no material has to be removed from the spinal canal. If you have spondylolisthesis or scoliosis, anterior fusion is a viable option. Anterior fusion is also the procedure used for the diagnoses involving discogenic pain (degenerative disc disease, black disc, IDD). Because I part company with surgeons who do *any* fusion for discogenic pain, though, I don't think that the type matters.

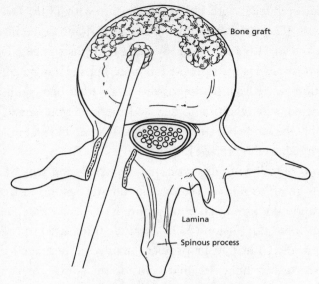

Transforaminal Lumbar Interbody Fusion (TLIF)

In a TLIF, the facet is removed, preserving the lamina and spinous process and the angled approach means nerves are not moved out of position.

> **Should I have an anterior or posterior fusion?** If you are confused, you are not alone. It's a complex decision, and your doctor will help you make it, but you should remember that deciding on the kind of fusion to have is not nearly as important as deciding whether you should have a fusion at all.

Circumferential fusions (the combination of front and back fusion) are done in one of two ways. One way is to do it through a TLIF or PLIF (both are circumferential); TLIFs fuse the vertebral

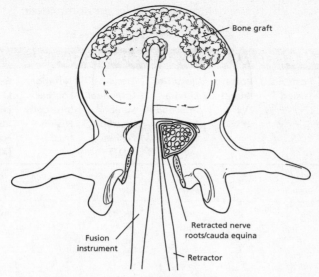

Bone graft

Retracted nerve
roots/cauda equina

Fusion
instrument

Retractor

Posterior Lumbar Interbody Fusion (PLIF)

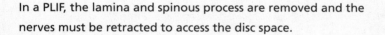

In a PLIF, the lamina and spinous process are removed and the
nerves must be retracted to access the disc space.

body, and can make use of the spinous process, the remaining
facet joint and the lamina that isn't removed (one gets removed
along with the facet), and PLIFs fuse the vertebral body, but can
also incorporate the facet joints, and the transverse process (the
spinous process and both laminae are removed). With either TLIF
or PLIF, the front and back portions of the surgery are done
through one incision. The other way is to do a "front-back" surgery where your surgeon opts instead to do the interbody portion
of the program from the front, and do the posterior portion from
a separate incision in the back. Again, all these options have advantages and disadvantages, and we don't have specific enough evidence to say that one way is safer than another.

I know all of this is complicated, so let me summarize:

WHAT GETS FUSED IN EACH OF THE FUSION PROCEDURES						
	Posterior Fusion (PF)	Postero-lateral Fusion (PLF)	Posterior Lumbar Interbody Fusion (PLIF)	Trans-foraminal Lumbar Interbody Fusion (TLIF)	Anterior Lumbar Interbody Fusion (ALIF)	Extreme Lateral Lumbar Interbody Fusion (XLIF)
Transverse Process	yes, if possible	yes	yes, if PLF done	yes, if PLF done	no	no
Facet Joint	yes	yes	yes, if PLF done	yes, if PF and/or PLF done	no	no
Spinous Process/ Lamina	yes	no	no	yes, if PF done	no	no
Interver-tebral Disc	no	no	yes	yes	yes	yes

Find the procedure you are considering in the top row and then look down the column to see what parts of the spine get fused for that procedure. NOTE: A PLIF or TLIF technically only describes interbody fusion, but in practice, many surgeons add a posterior fusion (PF) or posterolateral fusion (PLF).

GOT HARDWARE? INSTRUMENTATION

There is one more choice when it comes to deciding on a type of fusion: to instrument or not to instrument. Instruments are the rods, wires, cages, screws, and various other implants that surgeons use to hold the bones together and in the right position while the fusion heals. In some cases, they're necessary. In others, they may increase the time the surgery takes, the risk of infection, of nerve damage, of bleeding, and the bill, all without increasing the chance that the fusion will succeed. Instrumentation is such an important issue that I've given it its own chapter (it's the one after this one). If you decide to get fusion surgery, you need to read that chapter. If you decide not to, you can skip it.

PUTTING IT ALL TOGETHER: WHICH FUSION FOR WHICH PROBLEM

Now that you know the conditions for which fusion is indicated, and the types of fusion, it's time to match the right surgery to the right condition. It's impossible for me to list definitively all the conditions for which fusion is appropriate and which kind of fusion is absolutely, positively, the right choice. This list can only give you an idea of the general uses of each variety.

Posterior (fusing the spinous process, laminae, and facets) is the simplest fusion procedure, but it is the least common because most fusion surgery requires the removal of the spinous process and laminae. An example of a posterior fusion is scoliosis surgery. Posterior fusion isn't an option for any surgery that requires access to the spinal canal, so it can't be used to treat spondylolisthesis with stenosis, or any other condition that requires a laminectomy along with the fusion. Many times, a posterior fusion is combined with a posterolateral fusion.

Posterolateral (fusing the transverse processes and facets) can be used for any kind of condition. In most cases, it's the simplest procedure with the lowest risk of complications, and unless there's compelling evidence that a more complicated fusion will have a better outcome, this is the surgery I go with.

PLIF (fusing the vertebral body, and, if possible, transverse processes and the facet joint) and TLIF (fusing the vertebral body, and, if possible the spinous process, and the one lamina and facet that aren't removed) are used for both primary and revision surgery (I explain why in chapter 18). They are also used for grades one and two spondylolisthesis despite the fact that posterolateral fusion has possibly better results.[xiii] If the spondylolisthesis is severe (more than a grade two), a posterolateral fusion is simpler and safer; there is no evidence that PLIFs or TLIFs get better results.

ALIF/XLIF (fusing the vertebral body alone) has many uses. It's good for scoliosis. Also, an anterior approach may be the best treatment for certain tumors and fractures, and some revision surgery, particularly for pseudarthrosis. It is also the approach used for disc replacement. Probably the number-one use of this procedure in the United States, however, is for discogenic low back pain, for which I don't think you should have fusion at all.

Matching the procedure to the problem is a judgment call, and different surgeons make different judgments. There's not a lot of hard data to go on. In a few cases, like spondylolisthesis, we have some research comparing the efficacy of different kinds of fusion, but, in most cases, we don't. If you've decided to get fusion surgery, you should talk to your surgeon about what kind she recommends, and why. Your surgeon's preference and expertise are important factors to take into consideration.

WHAT CAN GO WRONG

Fusion is risky surgery, and that makes some decisions easier and some harder. If you're considering fusion for discogenic back pain, and I haven't talked you out of it already, this section might just make your decision easier. When you're weighing serious risks against dubious benefits, the answer should be obvious.

If you're considering fusion for one of the destabilizing conditions, this section may make your decision harder. The benefits may be significant, but they are by no means certain, and you have to weigh that uncertainty against these risks. This is the kind of difficult decision I walk my patients through every day. It's a hard decision, and it's made harder by the difficulty of pinning down complication rates. They vary by condition, they vary by study, they vary by doctor.

All fusion, though, has significant risks; one of the studies on fusion for back pain found that at least 18 percent of patients had complications within two weeks and another 6 percent had complications after two weeks,[xiv] but other studies say other things. (Instrumented fusions in general and instrumented circumferential fusions in particular are the riskiest kinds, and I cover those risks in the next chapter.) The best I can do is describe the possibilities and give you some idea of whether the chance they'll happen to you is small or large.

The risks I cover here are the long-term risks of fusion. There are also surgical complications, such as spinal fluid leaks, nerve damage, and blood vessel injury, which are covered in chapter 17: General Complications. Make sure you read that chapter before you make a decision about surgery.

When you consider what can go wrong with fusion surgery, you have to keep in mind that the risk of complications is not the same as the risk that the surgery won't solve your problem. It's certainly possible that you can have a complication-free surgery and a quick recovery but leave the hospital with the same problem you were admitted with.

FUSION NON-UNION

A fusion non-union, also called pseudarthrosis ("false joint"), happens when the bones don't knit together to form that one inflexible unit. I've already mentioned that fusions don't always fuse; in fact, it's safe to say that they often don't fuse. Estimates of pseudarthrosis run as high as 55 percent.[xv] Circumferential fusions are more likely to fuse than other kinds,[xvi] and interbody fusions are more likely to fuse than posterior. Surprisingly, it's not always easy to tell whether a fusion takes, because radiologic tests don't make it clear.

You can get a non-union in any kind of broken bone, and we're pretty serious about fixing them in the long bones. If you have a non-union in your femur, you've got trouble. Not necessarily so in the spine. What's interesting about fusion non-union is that it sometimes doesn't seem to matter.

> **Pseudarthrosis is not as scary as it sounds:** Studies show that pseudarthrosis, or non-union of a surgical fusion, can occur up to 50 percent of the time. Surprisingly, in most patients, it doesn't seem to be a problem. This is one of the great mysteries of spinal fusion surgery.

Often, and for a variety of conditions, patients whose fusions don't fuse do just about as well as patients whose fusions do fuse. Not only is this true for fusion surgery done for low back pain,[xvii] it's also true when fusion is done for some of the conditions that cause instability.[xviii] The question of why is one of the enigmas of spine surgery. If the point of the procedure is to immobilize a segment that's causing pain or instability, why would the patient who ended up with a pseudarthrosis do as well as the one whose fusion took?

We can speculate, particularly on the question of fusion for low back pain. When the disc is removed, that might relieve at least some of the pain, regardless of whether the vertebrae above and below are successfully immobilized. It's possible that the disc itself was painful, and movement didn't have much to do with it. Some doctors also posit that there's some reduction in motion even in pseudarthrosis. (They call this a fibrous union since scar and granulation tissue may provide for some stability.) A third theory is that it's likely that fusion doesn't work for back pain at all, so it doesn't matter whether the fusion fuses or not. There may be some truth in all of these theories.

Regardless of the original reason you had a fusion surgery, a non-union is an issue only if it causes pain, instability, deformity, or risks nerve damage. In that case, you may have to undergo a second fusion. The likelihood of the necessity for a revision procedure varies so much that it's impossible to predict. It depends on your original problem, as well as what kind of fusion you got, and technical issues regarding the surgery. Unfortunately, a second fusion can be a riskier undertaking than a first (see chapter 17).

There are several factors that increase the risk for non-union. First is the number of vertebrae being fused; the more you're fusing, the higher the risk. Second is the type of bone graft (which I describe in detail in the section on bone grafts at the end of this chapter). Third is the presence and nature of implants (see chapter 14). Fourth is smoking, which you absolutely, positively shouldn't do if you want your fusion to take. Fifth is drugs. There are some medications that impede fusion, the most common of which are nonsteroidal anti-inflammatories and some osteoporosis medications.

There are two strategies, bracing and stimulation, that doctors employ to encourage union, but neither has been well studied. Doctors use them because they intuitively feel they might help, and they do it with the best of intentions, but there's no evidence that either is effective.

Bracing limits motion, and it's appealing to believe that limiting motion would be conducive to fusion, in the same way you'd put a cast on a broken arm. Although long-term bracing can have serious consequences, short-term bracing has very little downside, and I discuss the advantages and disadvantages with my fusion patients.

There are also devices called stimulators that are supposed to increase the chance of a fusion's taking by bombarding it with magnetic or electrical impulses (or both). Stimulators come in internal and external varieties. The internal kind is implanted in your body next to the site of the fusion and the external kind is worn outside the body. If stimulation worked at all, the internal kind would probably have a better chance of helping your fusion fuse, but internal implantation also increases the odds of infection so much that I don't use internal stimulators. External stimulators have no downside other than cost and inconvenience, and I do sometimes use them.

Even if you jump through all the hoops, and your fusion fuses, there's no guarantee that your problem is solved. One study that looked at circumferential fusion for degenerative disc disease got the astonishingly high rate of fusion of 100 percent but nevertheless declared 50 percent of their procedures a failure because they didn't relieve the patients' pain.[xix] One commentator on the study concluded that "pseudarthrosis does not appear to be the dreaded complication that is often portrayed" and that "the obtainment of a solid fusion is in no way related to providing the patient with a reliable surgical solution."[xx]

ADJACENT LEVEL DISEASE/ADJACENT SEGMENT DISEASE

This is one of the most common problems with fusion surgery and also one of the most poorly studied. Adjacent level disease is another medical term that sounds complicated but is actually simple. Adjacent level disease is a problem in the motion segment (the combination of the disc and the vertebra next to it) above or below the vertebrae you had fused. It's not surprising that people have this problem, since fusing two vertebrae necessarily puts more stress on the vertebrae above and below.

To see why, I want you to visualize a train with four cars. A four-car train has three couplings and, if the train turns a corner, each coupling will account for one-third of the bend. Now picture a fusion of the center coupling into one long, immobile link. Now there are only two moveable couplings and, if the train turns the same amount as before, each coupling has to account for one-half the bend, significantly more than they did before the fusion.

The same things happen to your spine, and that extra bend is part of what makes fused spines vulnerable to the many problems that adjacent level disease can cause. The list of those problems is long, and includes spondylolisthesis, herniated discs, stenosis, facet arthritis, scoliosis, and compression fractures, as well as the all-purpose "instability."[xxi] How often those problems arise, and how serious they are, is a matter of some debate. There have been many studies, and the numbers are all over the map. An overview of the research found that the incidence of radiologic problems (such as disc degeneration, spondylolisthesis, bone spurs, and spinal stenosis) could be as high as 100 percent, and the incidence of problems that caused symptoms was in the 5–18 percent range.[xxii] In one 2003 study that followed patients for at least five years, 40 percent developed adjacent level "alterations," and half of those 40 percent had to get revision surgery.[xxiii] Suffice it to say that the numbers are large enough for you to take this risk very seriously.

Several factors increase the risk for adjacent level disease. The most obvious is the number of levels fused, but others are age (older is riskier), gender (women are at higher risk), osteoporosis (which weakens bone), and postmenopausal status (which puts you at risk for osteoporosis). One last risk, which I describe in the next chapter, is pedicle screws. If your doctor uses them, you're at higher risk for problems in adjacent levels.

FIXED SAGITTAL PLANE DEFORMITY (FSPD, A.K.A. FLATBACK SYNDROME)

This is a condition in which the lumbar spine has lost its normal swayback (or lordosis). In rare cases, it can occur as a complication of fusion. It was originally described as flatback deformity when it was associated with the use of Harrington rods for scoliosis surgery. FSPD can be the result of several different conditions, including fracture, trauma, and disc degeneration (see chapter 7: The Usual Suspects).

BONE GRAFTING

When two vertebrae are fused together, something has to be put either between or alongside them. The role of that something is twofold. First, it's to make sure that height and alignment are preserved (or restored, if either has been lost). Second, it's to facilitate the fusing of the two vertebrae into one inflexible unit. The most common something is a bone graft.

There are two sources of bone for a bone graft: you, or somebody else. If the graft comes from you, it's called (for obvious reasons) an autograft, and it's the best choice. Bone harvested from your own body is alive and therefore the most likely to promote the bone growth that's necessary for fusion. There is no risk that you are going to reject it or pick up an infection from it. The disadvantage, of course, is that the bone has to come from somewhere in your body. If you're having a laminectomy to go with your fusion, the removed laminae and spinous process is the obvious candidate for your graft. If you're not having a laminectomy, or if the bone removed isn't big enough to fill the gap between the vertebrae, you're going to have to get bone from someplace else.

The usual someplace else is the iliac crest. It's what you probably think of as your hip bone, but it is actually your pelvis. It's a big bone and can afford to give some of itself up for a graft. Harvesting it, though, has risks of its own. For starters, it hurts. It also often requires another incision, which means another risk of infection, nerve damage, and hematoma. The gluteus muscles have to be stripped off the bone, and this can cause muscle weakening. In the worst case, if your doctor takes too much bone, you could end up with a broken pelvis (this is rare). Another site that is sometimes used for a bone graft is the ribs. If you're having an anterior fusion, your surgeon can nip off a piece of one of them on her way in.

You can avoid all of these problems—but encounter a new set—by getting a bone graft from somebody else (an allograft), and there are bone banks that facilitate that. (Yes, they get their bones from dead people.) There are two kinds of allografts: whole bone, and demineralized bone matrix, which is essentially bone mush that's had all the minerals removed. The biggest problem with any allograft is that it's not as good as an autograft at stimulating bone growth. You can also pick up an infection from donated bone, although that's very rare.

There are also a group of synthetic bone graft substitutes made out of a variety of substances, including coral, collagen, ceramic, and biodegradable polymers. They're cheap, don't cause infections, and the supply is plentiful; but they don't work as well as autografts.

There is a promising new alternative: chemicals, specifically in the form of bone morphogenic proteins (BMP). BMPs are molecules that your body uses to form new bone. Many of them have been isolated and are now being genetically manufactured. As of this writing, there is only one that is FDA-approved (although others are being investigated), and it's only approved for anterior lumbar surgery. It has the catchy name of rhBMP-2, and I believe it is the future of bone grafting. It stimulates bone growth (even without a graft), and so avoids all of the risks that come with bone grafts. Once we get the kinks worked out, BMP may change the way spinal fusion is done.

The bone graft choice is a complicated one, and I've only scratched the surface here. I want you to know what the choices are, but one of the biggest considerations is what kind of graft your surgeon prefers. Different doctors like to use different materials, and your doctor's comfort level may outweigh other concerns when it comes to bone graft material. Work with your doctor to make the choice.

RECOVERY

Fusion is major surgery. You'll probably be in the hospital three to five days, but you should be out of bed the day after the procedure. You can expect considerable pain for several days, and I always discuss the advantages and disadvantages of patient-controlled anesthesia (PCA)—a pain pump. In any case, the pain should start to subside quickly, within twenty-four to forty-eight hours.

Once you're home, I advise you to avoid lifting, twisting, or bending, but I'm strongly in favor of walking. The time it takes to recover completely varies dramatically. I've had patients who are 100 percent within a couple of months. Others take much longer, or never get there at all.

Recovery also varies by the type of fusion you've had. It's easier to recover from anterior fusion because there's no muscle damage. Posterior recovery takes longer. It's also easier to recover from a one-level fusion than a multilevel fusion, and, as always, it's easier to recover when you're young.

ENDNOTES

i R. A. Deyo, et al., "United States Trends in Lumbar Fusion Surgery for Degenerative Conditions," *Spine* 30, no. 12 (2005), pp. 1441–45.

ii S. D. Boden, "Overview of the Biology of Lumbar Spine Fusion and Principles for Selecting a Bone Graft Substitute," *Spine* 27, no. 16s (2002), pp. S26–31.

iii R. A. Deyo, A. Nachemson, S. K. Mirza, "Spinal-Fusion Surgery—The Case for Restraint," *New England Journal of Medicine* 350, no. 7 (2004), pp. 722–26.

iv A. White and M. Panjabi, *Clinical Biomechanics of the Spine*, 2nd ed. (Philadelphia: J. B. Lippincott, 1990), p. 278.

v J. M. Muggleton, M. Kondracki, R. Allen, "Spinal Fusion for Lumbar Instability: Does It Have a Scientific Basis?," *Journal of Spinal Disorders* 13, no. 3 (2000), pp. 200–4.

E. N. Hanley, "The Indications for Lumbar Spinal Fusion with and Without Instrumentation," *Spine* 20, no. 24s (1995), pp. 143s–53s.

vi P. J. Slosar, "Indications and Outcomes of Reconstructive Surgery in Chronic Pain of Spinal Origin," *Spine* 27, no. 22 (2002), pp. 2555–62.

vii P. Fritzell, et al., "2001 Volvo Award Winner in Clinical Studies: Lumbar Fusion *Versus* Nonsurgical Treatment for Chronic Low Back Pain: A Multicenter Randomized Controlled Trial from the Swedish Lumbar Spine Study Group," *Spine* 26, no. 23 (2001), pp. 2521–32.

viii Ibid.

ix J. I. Brox, et al., "Randomized Clinical Trial of Lumbar Instrumented Fusion and Cognitive Intervention and Exercises in Patients with Chronic Low Back Pain and Disc Degeneration," *Spine* 28, no. 17 (2003), pp. 1913–21.

x J. Fairbank, et al., "Randomised Controlled Trial to Compare Surgical Stabilisation of the Lumbar Spine with an Intensive Rehabilitation Programme for Patients with Chronic Low Back Pain: The MRC Spine Stabilisation Trial," *British Medical Journal* 330, (2005), p. 1233–39.

xi J.N.A. Gibson, G. Waddell, "Surgery for Degenerative Lumbar Spondylosis: updated Cochrane Review," *Spine* 30, no. 20 (2005), pp. 2312–20.

xii R. A. Deyo, et al., "Spinal-Fusion Surgery—The Case for Restraint."

xiii S. Madan, N. R. Boeree, "Outcome of Posterior Lumbar Interbody Fusion *Versus* Posterolateral Fusion for Spondylolytic Spondylolisthesis," *Spine* 27, no. 14 (2002), pp. 1536–42.

xiv P. Fritzell, et al., "2001 Volvo Award Winner."

xv J. S. Fischgrund, et al., "1997 Volvo Award Winner in Clinical Studies: Degenerative Lumbar Spondylolisthesis with Spinal Stenosis: A Prospective, Randomized Study Comparing Decompressive Laminectomy and Arthrodesis with and Without Spinal Instrumentation," *Spine* 22, no. 24 (1997), pp. 2807–12.

xvi S. D. Gertzbein, M. R. Hollopeter, S. Hall, "Pseudarthrosis of the Lumbar Spine: Outcome after Circumferential Fusion," *Spine* 23, no. 21 (1998), pp. 2352–56.

xvii P. Fritzell, et al., "2001 Volvo Award Winner."

xviii H. N. Herkowitz, L. T. Kurz, "Degenerative Lumbar Spondylolisthesis with Spinal Stenosis: A Prospective Study Comparing Decompression with Decompression and Intertransverse Process Arthrodesis," *Journal of Bone and Joint Surgery (Am.)* 73, no. 6 (1991), pp. 802–08.

xix S. D. Gertzbein, et al., "Pseudarthrosis of the Lumbar Spine."

xx H. N. Herkowitz, et al., "Point of View: Pseudarthrosis of the Lumbar Spine: Outcome After Circumferential Fusion," *Spine* 23, no. 2 (1998), pp. 2356–57.

xxi P. Park, et al., "Adjacent Segment Disease After Lumbar or Lumbosacral Fusion: Review of the Literature," *Spine* 29, no. 17 (2004), pp. 1938–44.

xxii Ibid.

xxiii P. Gillet, "The Fate of the Adjacent Motion Segments After Lumbar Fusion," *Journal of Spinal Disorders & Techniques* 16, no. 4 (2003), pp. 338–45.

Chapter 14

SPINAL IMPLANTS

S pinal implants are the rods, hooks, wires, cages, and screws that doctors install in your body during surgery to hold your spine in a particular position after a spinal fusion. They're also called instrumentation, or hardware. Hardware is a fitting name for it, since most of it looks a lot like the stuff you find in the bins at Home Depot. It's higher-tech, though, and a lot more expensive.

Technically, bone grafts and bone cement, which I mention in other chapters, are also implants, as is anything else you put in the human body. But here we're going to talk specifically about fusion-related implants other than bone grafts. It's these implants that define the difference between an instrumented and noninstrumented fusion, and it's these implants that you may have to make difficult decisions about. Introducing foreign bodies into human bodies raises the risk of complications of any surgery. They can be placed in a wrong position, break, loosen, and get infected.

The reason to get fusion-related implants is twofold. They provide interim stability and alignment while the fusion heals, and they facilitate that healing. Both make intuitive sense. If I'm operating on a patient to stabilize a painful, unstable spine, the rods

I implant keep the painful parts from moving around in the several months required for the fusion to take. At the same time, they facilitate that fusion precisely because they minimize motion, thereby increasing the odds that the graft will be successful. They act as a kind of clamp. Think about gluing two pieces of wood together; you don't just apply the glue and walk away. You put the pieces in a clamp so they can't move while the glue dries overnight. In the same way, the implants clamp the bones together while the fusion takes—although it won't happen overnight.

There is very little disagreement about those two functions. There's ample evidence that implants do provide interim stability and do facilitate fusion, although it's difficult to determine the extent to which they do it. And while a speedy recovery is important, the critical issue about implants is that second function—facilitating fusion.

In the previous chapter I mentioned that a patient whose fusion takes often doesn't have a better outcome than a patient whose fusion doesn't. For many conditions, the chances of pain relief and improved function are the same whether or not you end up with a pseudarthrosis. I know that it's difficult to come to terms with the idea that it doesn't matter whether your fusion fuses or not, but in many cases it's true.

So the question of whether to use implants boils down to this: will *your* outcome be better if your fusion fuses solid? If the answer is no, then there's no reason to get an instrumented fusion. If the answer is yes, then you have to weigh that advantage against the risks of adding implants to the surgery.

There are times when the advantages resoundingly outweigh the risks. If your spine comes apart as a result of a traumatic injury, a successful fusion is critical, and implants are the only way we can keep the bones together while the fusion heals. In fusion for scoliosis surgery, the implants align the spine until the bones fuse in their new position.

Because I am extremely cautious in recommending fusion surgery to my patients—and to my readers—I think that the implant decision is often simple. Most of the controversy about implants relates to the question of whether they should be used in fusion for discogenic low back pain. Since I don't think that you should have fusion for discogenic pain diagnoses, the question of implants is moot.

Most of the conditions for which I do fusion surgery are the very conditions for which it matters that the fusion fuses (fracture, trauma, scoliosis, spondylolisthesis), and so most of my fusions are instrumented. The exception is spondylolisthesis, for which I have strict criteria that determine whether I use instruments or not.

Let me sum up my take on implants in one paragraph. If you're having a fusion for any of the destabilizing conditions I discussed in the previous chapter, other than spondylolisthesis, implants are likely to improve your outcome. If you're getting it for spondylolisthesis, implants are appropriate in some cases and inappropriate in others. If you're getting a fusion for one of the discogenic pain diagnoses, you shouldn't be getting implants because you shouldn't be having surgery at all.

Now let me explain in a little more detail.

TYPES OF IMPLANTS

If you're facing the "to instrument or not to instrument" question, you need to start by understanding exactly what implants are. There are two basic kinds: connectors and spacers. Connectors are usually used to keep the spine from moving while a spinal fusion fuses—the clamp function—and they take the form of rods, wires, cables, hooks, and screws. Spacers serve the opposite function. When vertebral bones have collapsed or discs have been removed, spacers, which can be made of bone, polymer, or metal, hold the bones above and below apart while the fusion heals. Some spacers are solid, some are rings, and some are cylinders (or rectangles) with holes in them—those are called cages. The newest kind of spacer is a disc replacement, which has a chapter all to itself.

If you're having the kind of procedure that removes an entire disc, you have to have a spacer put in to keep the two vertebrae from rubbing together. If you're getting an interbody fusion, the decision you and your doctor have to make is what kind of spacer to use, not whether to use one. The different kinds have different advantages and different risks, but there's not a lot of research comparing them. I'm not going to give you a detailed comparison because I think the advantage of going with the kind your surgeon prefers and is accustomed to outweighs any advantage you might get from asking her to switch. If you're concerned about spacers, the discussion you should be having with your doctor is why you're having the kind of surgery that requires them.

When we speak of an instrumented fusion, however, we're generally not talking about spacers. In common parlance, it's the connectors—primarily rods and screws—that make a fusion instrumented. There's no formal definition of "instrumented," but this is the way I hear it used most often, and the way I use it in this book. Unlike spacers, connectors are often optional, and they're the implants around which the controversy centers.

Connectors need to be strong, and so they're all made of metal, either stainless steel or titanium. Stainless steel was the material of choice for a long time, but in many instances titanium is used because steel interferes with both MRI and CT scan images. The metal doesn't prevent you from having either scan, but the results are often unreadable. Titanium, though, is MRI-compatible (but, like stainless steel, interferes with CT), and is easier to work with than steel because it isn't as stiff.

The perfect connector would be strong enough to hold your bones together while your fusion healed, not interfere with any tests or scans, and be harmlessly absorbed by your body once your spine is solid. We don't have it yet, but that's the direction implant research is taking. There are such implants in other fields of surgery, and it's probably only a matter of time before the technology gets to the point that we can make them for backs.

More important than what connectors are made of is what they do, and how they do it. In order to clamp your bones together while your fusion fuses, the hardware has to physically attach to your spine. This attachment point is where most implant trouble originates.

The part of the vertebra in which we anchor screws is the pedicle, the bone that connects the front of the vertebra to the back. (Take a minute to flip back to page 7; knowing exactly where the pedicle is will help you understand this chapter.) The most commonly used anchors are screws called pedicle screws, and they're screwed directly into the pedicle. If a screw is put in the right place, the pedicle can support it without a problem. If it's a little too far to one side, though, or a little too deep, you can have damage to nerves and vessels. Hooks and wires are alternatives to pedicle screws, but they're being used less and less frequently because screws provide a much more solid anchor.

> **Spinal implants: do you really need one?** Having a spinal fusion doesn't necessarily mean you have to have an implant. Implants carry their own risks and benefits, and the decision to use them should be considered separately from the decision to have a fusion.

Now that you know what implants are, and how they work, let's go back to what they can do.

WHAT IMPLANTS ARE GOOD FOR

As I explained at the beginning of this chapter, implants matter if it is important that your bones stay in alignment while the fusion heals, or, if your bones are aligned, that your fusion takes. In the previous chapter, I listed the conditions for which fusion has a long track record of fusing successfully. The list of conditions for which a successful fusion is important is very similar. There's only one item on the list—spondylolisthesis—for which implants may or may not be necessary. I'm going to cover the easy categories first, and then discuss spondylolisthesis at some length.

Before you read about the conditions for which implants are used, I want to remind you that there are some kinds of fusion that are almost always instrumented, no matter what underlying condition they're treating. All TLIFs are instrumented because the procedure requires the removal of one of the facets. That's enough to make a spine unstable, and so rods and pedicle screws are necessary to facilitate fusion. Most, but not all, PLIFs are also instrumented, for the same reason. The amount of bone removed in a PLIF varies, but it's generally enough to risk destabilization if the fusion doesn't fuse. If you're getting one of those procedures, you need to understand why your surgeon has chosen it over a kind of fusion that doesn't require instrumentation. If, however, you're getting a posterolateral fusion, posterior fusion, or ALIF (which requires a spacer), the instrumentation decision needs to be made based on your condition.

Tumor, fracture, infection, scoliosis, kyphosis: If you're getting fusion for any of these, implants are probably indicated. Remember that having one of these conditions doesn't automatically mean you need surgery, but if what you have is severe enough to need the fusion, you're probably going to have to make it an instrumented fusion.

Any of these conditions can cause instability, neurological damage, deformity, and pain. Implants both support the weakened spine as it heals and help ensure that the fusion will take. And, if you have any of these conditions, it's important to minimize the chance of the fusion failing to take.

Revision surgery: There are many reasons you may need a second surgery, and many of them call for instrumentation. I cover revision surgery case by case in chapter 18.

Spondylolisthesis: This is the hard one. The evidence for instrumentation improving the outcome for spondylolisthesis isn't conclusive. In fact, it's all over the map. I think there are cases for which instrumentation is needed, and many more for which it isn't.

It would be easy to believe that instrumentation always helps a spondylolisthesis patient. The vertebra has slipped forward, and it seems that a solid fusion would be critical to successful recovery. It turns out, though, that there's contradictory evidence to support that conclusion.

One of the first prospective, randomized studies on the issue was done back in 1993, and it *did* support that conclusion; it found that instrumentation did indeed improve patient outcomes.[i] Nevertheless, a meta-analysis published the following year found no statistical difference between the outcomes for patients with spondylolisthesis who had fusion surgery with and without instrumentation.[ii] The analysis necessarily included research that wasn't randomized or prospective, and it's always tricky to draw solid conclusions from suboptimal data. If a whole bunch of flawed studies all find that instrumented fusion isn't better, though, the topic deserves another look.

From 1997 to 2000 three well-recognized and well-performed studies took that look, and all found that instrumentation didn't improve outcomes.[iii] Interestingly, one of these studies[iv] showed that the fusion rate was *higher* in uninstrumented surgery (85 percent) than in instrumented fusion surgery (68 percent) but the difference was not considered statistically significant.

Several years later, though, the researchers on one of those studies followed up with a group of the patients from the original study.[v] They only followed up with the noninstrumented fusion group, so we can't compare instrumented to noninstrumented outcomes. What they found, though, was that at an average follow-up of seven years, eight months, the patients who had a solid fusion did have less pain and were able to be more active than those who had a pseudarthrosis.[vi]

A medical review for spine doctors published in 2005 sums up my assessment of fusion for spondylolisthesis: "Lumbar arthrodesis has been shown to be of clear benefit in reducing pain and improving function. But because of the conflicting reports in the literature, the merits of supplemental instrumentation are not as clear. Instrumentation seems to increase fusion rates and likely prevents progression of spondylolisthesis, but has not been definitively shown to improve clinical outcome."[vii]

I use instrumentation in some, but not all, cases of spondylolisthesis. First, if a patient has definitive radiographic instability (significant slippage of one bone on another or abnormal motion between two bones—both of which are seen on an X-ray), I think it's likely that a solid fusion may have a better long-term outcome. The generally accepted radiographic criteria for instability are seen on radiographs and include more than ten degrees of angulation or at least four millimeters of slippage with flexion and extension. My concern is that the spondylolisthesis will slip further following laminectomy surgery or that the slipped bones will fuse in the worst position. Second is the presence of severe spondylolisthesis (grade three or above). Third is the presence of an associated deformity (like scoliosis). There are other reasons I can think of, but in the absence of good data, all I have to rely on is my clinical experience and best judgment. So will your doctor.

Whether or not to use implants isn't the only important question if you're getting fusion for spondylolisthesis. You also have to decide about the kind of fusion. I prefer a posterolateral fusion—the simplest kind. Many doctors, though, have begun to do PLIFs and TLIFs (see page 219 for a refresher), which are more complicated versions of fusion. The evidence is that a straightforward (and less risky) posterolateral fusion is just as effective and a lot safer. If your doctor is recommending a PLIF or TLIF, you should talk to him about the reasons for his decision.[viii]

WHAT IMPLANTS ARE NOT GOOD FOR

In two words: everything else.

I want to start this section by stating the obvious: If a fusion is inappropriate, an instrumented fusion is *really* inappropriate.

The list of conditions for which instrumented fusion is appropriate is almost identical to the list of conditions for which fusion is appropriate. What's left to include in this section is those conditions that fusion, instrumented or not, shouldn't be used to treat. At the top of that list is discogenic pain, which is increasingly being treated with instrumented fusion. As you know, I think fusion for chronic back pain is suspect, but I recognize that you may not take my word for it. If you disagree, you may have decided to get fused despite my best persuasive efforts. Since I didn't convince you not to get fusion, it is unlikely that I can convince you not to get an instrumented fusion, but I'll give it my best shot.

I'll give you the executive summary first. Patients who get instrumented fusions for their back pain don't do any better than patients who get noninstrumented fusions. Whether or not your fusion takes doesn't seem to matter to your recovery.

Ironically, it's the favorite study of fusion-for-back-pain advocates that offers the last word on instrumented fusion for back pain. Remember the 2001 study I talked about in chapter 13 that found that fusion did help back pain? (If you don't, it's on page 212.) The authors did a follow-up study in 2002, and compared those subjects who had gotten a simple posterolateral fusion to those who had gotten either posterolateral fusion with instrumentation or a circumferential fusion with instrumentation. The patients who got the simplest procedure, the noninstrumented posterolateral fusion, did as well as the others for both pain reduction and overall outcome. This is true despite different fusion rates (72 percent of the posterolateral fusions fused, compared to 87 percent of the instrumented posterolateral fusions and 91 percent of the circumferential fusions). This fact didn't escape the authors' notice. "A disturbing finding," they wrote, "which the authors share with others, is that there was no correlation between an osseous fusion and a positive patient rating."[ix] (An osseous fusion is one that fused.) There you have it, straight from the horse's mouth. Even the people who believe in fusion for back pain don't support the use of instrumentation. They're in good company there. There's other research that concludes the same thing. But I think the fact that even true believers in fusion for discogenic pain don't advocate implants is very compelling.

There's one last reason not to get implants, and that's if you have a condition that is a contraindication. If you have osteoporosis, your bones may be too soft to hold the implant.

If you have an active infection or an allergy to one of the materials the implants are made of, make sure that your doctor knows; it may preclude surgery unless you're getting it for a life-threatening condition.

RESEARCH SUMMARY OF IMPLANTS

- If you're having fusion for a tumor, fracture, or infection, or for scoliosis or kyphosis, instrumentation is important to the success of the surgery.
- Implants for spondylolisthesis should be made on a case-by-case basis.
- Instrumentation does not necessarily improve outcomes in fusion for back pain.
- The use of instrumentation raises the risk of both short-term and long-term complications.

WHAT CAN GO WRONG

Fusion surgery with implants is relatively risky. You have all of the risks of fusion, which I talked about in the previous chapter, plus the added risks of implants. Remember the Swedish study I just talked about? They reviewed the early complication rates for the different types of surgery they compared. Their results were startling: 6 percent for posterolateral fusion, 16 percent for posterolateral fusion with instrumentation, and 31 percent in the "circumferential fusion."[x]

The risks fall into two categories. Instrumented fusion surgery itself is longer and more complicated than noninstrumented fusion, and so more can go wrong on the table, and in the immediate aftermath. Beyond that, there are long-term risks associated with having the implants in your body.

Surgery risks: There is always the chance of something going wrong during the procedure itself, or just afterwards. Complications are related to so many variables that it's almost impossible to give hard data for each of them. I don't think that any two studies of the complications of implants have ever gotten identical results. Specific complications include (but are not limited to) wrong site surgery, infected implants, spinal fluid leak, nerve damage (temporary or permanent), broken and/or dislodged implants, and painful hardware. Many people also don't appreciate the importance of related factors that also affect the chance of a complication with implants. These include your overall health, the quality/strength of your bone, a history of smoking, whether you are having primary or revision surgery, the approach (from the front or back), whether a laminectomy is also being carried out with your implant placement, the type of implant and a whole host of other factors that are too numerous to list.

Prior to surgery, spend the extra time to discuss these and other important issues with your surgeon. What I want you to take away from this section is not that you have a 1–2 percent chance of a deep tissue infection; it's that the odds of having a complication of one kind or another are real. Do not get an instrumented fusion unless the benefits are commensurately significant.

Long-term risks: I already mentioned that spacers carry risks. They can subside (which means they sink into the bone), they can slip out of place, and they can get infected. If you're getting an interbody fusion, though, you have to have a spacer, so I'm just going to leave it at that. The real issue here is the risks of the rods and pedicle screws that anchor them.

Out-of-position implants can happen in two ways: either your surgeon can put them in the wrong place or they can shift after the surgery. This is a particular danger with pedicle screws. The screw should go from the back of the vertebra, through the pedicle, and end in the vertebral body. A misplaced screw can end up in the spinal canal or neural foramen; in both places, nerve damage is a possibility. This is more likely than you might think; the spinal nerves and the cauda equina are only about a millimeter from the edge of the pedicle, and that doesn't leave much room for error. If the screws go in a little crooked, the consequences can be devastating. If you've ever tried to screw a screw straight into a piece of wood and had it go in at an angle, you know how easily that can happen. Putting in pedicle screws isn't much different. This is why your surgeon may choose to also monitor your nerves during surgery. With the use of special equipment, electrical impulses help detect whether nerves have been breeched. You may hear this referred to as intra-operative EMG or spinal cord monitoring. It is not fool-proof, however, and not all surgeons feel it is necessary.

Properly placed or not, a screw can pull out of the bone, particularly if the bone has been softened by age, osteoporosis, illness, steroids, infection, or a lifetime of insufficient calcium. When this happens, you lose the anchor for the implant, and therefore the stability of the structure.

If you end up with an out-of-position implant, the treatment for it depends on just how out of position it is. If it threatens damage, it has to be removed. If it's not doing it's job, ditto. Sometimes, if neither is the case, the implants don't need to come out. The decision is usually made on a case-by-case basis.

CASE STUDY

FRANK is a twenty-five-year-old man who came to me with severe low back pain. He had been suffering with back problems since his teens. He knew he had a "slipped bone" in his back as an adolescent. Recently, the pain began to get worse and was now affecting his ability to stand at work as a salesman. He could no longer play sports because of the pain. He had recently developed severe sciatica. Tests revealed a grade two spondylolisthesis at L5-S1 and a large herniated disc severely compressing the nerves. To make matters worse, the flexion and extension X-rays showed significant movement of the spondylolisthesis. He tried all of the alternative treatments and failed to improve his pain. We discussed surgery, which included a laminectomy to remove the herniated disc (for the sciatica) and a fusion from L5 to S1 with pedicle screws (for the spondylolisthesis). The reason I felt that the pedicle screws were important in this surgery was the unstable nature of the spondylolisthesis. The surgery went smoothly. Even the intra-operative spinal cord monitoring that I routinely use during this type of surgery showed no abnormalities. And yet, when he woke up in the operating room, he had a drop foot on one side. One of the pedicle screws was pressing on a nerve, and was immediately removed in a second procedure. It took six months, and a lot of physical therapy, but the strength in the foot finally came back to normal. The good news is that his sciatica is gone, as is his back pain, and he is back to enjoying his life.

Broken implants, unlike out-of-position implants, are usually a longer-term complication. As with out-of-position implants, the need to do something about them depends on the situation.

If you're wondering how something as sturdy as a metal rod can break just from your normal movement, think back to the last boring meeting you sat through, bending a paper clip back and forth until it snapped. The same phenomenon can happen in your back. The stress you put on an implant each time you bend over might not be much, but it's the same stress over and over. Eventually, the implant may give way.

What should you do about it? That depends on whether the broken implant is discovered before or after your fusion fuses. Hardware usually breaks because a fusion hasn't fused yet. The motion causes the paper clip phenomenon, and if it goes on long enough, just about any implant will break. After instrumented surgery, there is a race between the fusion taking and the implant failing. Will the fusion take before the implant breaks? Once the fusion takes, the implants are no longer under stress and are very unlikely to break, and the race is won.

If you find the broken hardware after a fusion has fused, it's a moot point. Your fusion has already healed and so, unless there's pain or the hardware is threatening a vital structure, the broken pieces can stay where they are.

If you find broken hardware before a fusion heals, it's a more difficult problem. Sometimes fusions will fuse despite the broken hardware. Other times they won't. If it's essential that your fusion take, or the broken hardware is causing a problem, you may have to undergo a revision procedure. Sometimes, though, even with an unfused fusion, further surgery isn't necessary.

There are things you can do to try to avoid broken implants. Make sure you follow your surgeon's postoperative instructions carefully. Don't smoke, since smokers are at higher risk for non-union, and therefore at higher risk for broken implants. And don't do anything dangerous, such as jumping out of trees or riding motorcycles, while your fusion is healing; if you hurt yourself, you might hurt your implants too.

Reoperation: All of these complications, both long and short term, can result in the need for another surgery. One study found that 25 percent of instrumented posterolateral fusions had to be revised, compared to 14 percent of noninstrumented fusions.[xi] There are many more studies with many more complication rates, but I want you to understand that the risk is very real, and very serious.

That's a scary list, and I want to assure you that, when used appropriately, implants play a vital role and their advantages significantly outweigh their disadvantages. I hope this chapter gave you a clear idea of the appropriate use of implants.

IMPLANTS, INDUSTRY, AND YOUR SURGEON

The decision to use implants is ideally made by you and your doctor. Often, though, there's a third party involved—the implant manufacturer. There are many different kinds of implants, each made by a different manufacturer vying for your doctor's business. You may have read newspaper articles about the lengths some of them have gone to in order to secure that business. The problems haven't been limited to implant manufacturers. Aggressive marketing tactics have raised eyebrows and prompted lawsuits in many areas of medicine where big money is at stake.

Fortunately, I think the implant industry is improving, and there aren't nearly as many aggressive tactics used now as there have been in past years.

I think it's important that implant manufacturers have adopted ethical and professional standards when dealing with doctors, because the industry-doctor partnership has to work. Industry needs doctors, and doctors need industry, to improve medicine. Manufacturers can't develop and fine-tune new products without feedback from doctors who use those products. Likewise, many of those products make doctors' jobs easier and medicine better.

Money isn't a guarantee that a doctor's judgment is compromised. I know excellent, conscientious doctors who earn consulting or speaking fees from implant manufacturers. But money can skew a doctor's judgment, and financial relationships between surgeons and industry is something I think patients need to be aware of.

There is always the possibility that your doctor has financial ties to the manufacturer of the implant being used in your surgery, and I believe your surgeon has an ethical obligation to disclose this information. Has he gotten any consulting fees or speaking honoraria? Does he receive research support? Does he have any financial stake in the company? Is he on the board of the company? Does he have stock or stock options? If the answer to any of these is yes, it doesn't necessarily mean that the choice to use implants, and those implants specifically, is wrong. It just means you should be aware of the issues, address them carefully, and discuss them with your surgeon.

ENDNOTES

i T. A. Zdeblick, "A Prospective, Randomized Study of Lumbar Fusion: Preliminary Results," *Spine* 18, no. 8 (1993), pp. 983–91.

ii S. M. Mardjetko, "Degenerative Lumbar Spondylolisthesis: A Meta-Analysis of the Literature 1970–1993," *Spine* 19, no. 20S (1994), pp. 2256S–65S.

iii J. S. Fischgrund, et al., "1997 Volvo Award Winner."

   K. Thomsen, et al., "1997 Volvo Award Winner in Clinical Studies: The Effect of Pedicle Screw Instrumentation on Functional Outcome and Fusion Rates in Posterolateral Lumbar Spinal Fusion: A Prospective, Randomized Clinical Study," *Spine* 22 (1997), pp. 2813–22.

   H. Möller, R. Hedlund, "Instrumented and Noninstrumented Posterolateral Fusion in Adult Spondylolisthesis: A Prospective Randomized Study: Part 2," *Spine* 25, no. 13 (2000), pp. 1716–21.

iv K. Thomsen, et al., "1997 Volvo Award Winner."

v H. N. Herkowitz, L. T. Kurz, "Degenerative Lumbar Spondylolisthesis with Spinal Stenosis," *Journal of Bone and Joint Surgery (Am.)* 73 (1991), p. 802–8.

vi M. B. Kornblum, et al., "Degenerative Lumbar Spondylolisthesis with Spinal Stenosis: A Prospective Long-term Study Comparing Fusion and Pseudarthrosis," *Spine* 29, no. 7 (2004), pp. 726–34.

vii J. C. Wang, et al., "Current Treatment Strategies for the Painful Lumbar Motion Segment: Posterolateral Fusion *Versus* Interbody Fusion," *Spine* 30, no. 16S (2005), pp. S33–S43.

viii S. Madan, N. R. Boeree, "Outcome of Posterior Lumbar Interbody Fusion."

ix P. Fritzell, et al., "Chronic Low Back Pain and Fusion: A Comparison of Three Surgical Techniques: A Prospective Multicenter Randomized Study from the Swedish Lumbar Spine Study Group," *Spine* 27, no. 11 (2002), pp. 1131–41.

x Ibid.

xi F. B. Christensen, E. S. Hansen, M. Laursen, et al., "Long-term Functional Outcome of Pedicle Screw Instrumentation as a Support for Posterolateral Spinal Fusion: Randomized Clinical Study with a 5-Year Follow-up," *Spine* 27, no. 12 (2002), pp. 1269–77.

Chapter 15

ARTIFICIAL DISC REPLACEMENT

The most recent innovation in back surgery, fresh from FDA approval in October 2004, is artificial disc replacement (ADR). The name says it all; it's a procedure to remove a suspected problem disc and insert a man-made replacement.

The surgery is similar to an anterior lumbar interbody fusion (ALIF). Your surgeon goes through your abdomen and removes the disc that's going to be replaced. Then he'll use special instruments to spread the bones apart to make room for the artificial disc. He'll slide the disc in, then remove the spreaders to bring the bones back together. The disc has little spikes on the top and bottom, and they keep the disc from slipping out of place in the same way that cleats give you traction on the soccer field. Once your spine is back together, the disc is supposed to perform just like the real thing.

We've gotten used to the idea that body parts can be replaced. Most of us have a parent or an aunt or a friend with an artificial knee or hip. Now discs have joined the list of replaceable parts. But, although comparing discs to knees and hips is understandable, it's not useful. The track record of disc replacement doesn't look anything like the excellent record of knee and hip replacement.

The artificial disc has been thirty years in the making. It's not easy to replicate the functions of the real thing. Compared to knees and hips, discs are complicated and the requirements for success are demanding. The discs you were born with have three basic functions: to allow for motion, to absorb shock, and to hold the bones of the spine together. The artificial disc has to do all those things, and is designed to mimic the real disc as closely as possible. It essentially consists of two metal plates with a plastic disc in between, a kind of spinal Oreo cookie.

WHY DISC REPLACEMENT?

The theory behind the claim that ADR can fix low back pain is similar to the one for the use of fusion for discogenic low back pain. If a disc is causing pain (and a variety of other criteria are met), you can stop the pain by decommissioning the disc. With fusion, that decommissioning happens by immobilizing the disc. With ADR, it happens by replacing the disc altogether.

According to its proponents, there are several advantages to ADR. The most important is that it preserves motion in the spine. In theory, it doesn't put adjacent discs at risk, both because there is no added stress from fusion and because the surgical procedure doesn't compromise the facet joints of the vertebrae above and below the replaced disc. Fusion does both of those things, which is why adjacent level disease is one of the major complications of fusion surgery. (If you want a refresher course on adjacent level disease, go back to chapter 13.)

There are a couple of other advantages that ADR may have over fusion. Because it's a less invasive procedure, patients are usually out of the hospital more quickly. There is nothing that has to fuse, there is no risk of non-union, and there is no period of restricted activity to give the bones time to knit together.

All in all, the theory sounds promising. As usual, though, the practice is much more complex. Early results indicate that some of the claims might pan out, while others probably won't. We don't yet have anything close to enough information to decide definitively whether ADR will be able to successfully treat back pain.

THE REALITY SO FAR

As with any other surgery, there are two basic questions. First, if the surgery itself goes off without a hitch (that is, with no significant complications), will it solve the problem (that is, fix the pain)? Second, what are the odds that the surgery goes off without a hitch?

Let's start with the first question—is ADR a good tool for alleviating low back pain? The answer is not likely. To get a more specific answer, let's look at the clinical trials so far. As I take you through them, it's important to remember that the patients in those trials are selected very carefully, and the surgeons are very well trained, so the research results must be read as a best-case scenario. Let's take a look at that best case.

While some studies conclude that the procedure can be very useful for some patients, it's important to consider their point of reference. Spinal fusion is the most frequently done procedure for low back pain, and is currently held up as the standard to which disc replacement is compared. The problem is that fusion in general, and the type of fusion the studies referenced in particular, is not a good standard; its results are mediocre, and many voices in the field, mine included, are asking hard questions about how and whether fusion works for pain.[i] Yet, if we look at the research, we find ADR being touted as a success if its results are similar to those achieved with fusion.

Research studies show that the early (less than two years) results of disc replacement are comparable and possibly better than that for fusion.[ii,iii] Patients are leaving the hospital sooner, they have less pain, and they are more functional. After two years, however, the results of the two procedures are similar. Stop for a moment and consider what this means. The people who have a lot invested in the success of this disc did clinical trials under optimal circumstances, with the most highly trained surgeons and the best-screened patients, with the result that the new technique didn't do any better (after two years) than the old technique, which is being widely questioned in the field.

WHAT CAN GO WRONG

Now we know the answer to the first question—whether ADR is effective in treating low back pain if the procedure goes well. Let's look at the odds that the procedure will go well. That's where the comparison to spinal fusion is even more telling. If a spinal fusion fuses properly, the most common complication, aside from the risk that the fusion doesn't stop the pain, is adjacent level disease, when problems develop in the areas of the spine above or below the fusion. Although we don't have comprehensive data, one study found that up to 40 percent of fusion patients had adjacent level "alterations" over the long term.[iv] At the risk of beating a dead horse, I want to emphasize that these are most definitely not good results. Fusion isn't good at fixing pain, and has a very high level of complications; when we evaluate ADR by comparing it to fusion on either front, we're starting with a bar that's very, very low.

As low as it is, I don't think the artificial disc gets over it. ADR has the conventional risks of any abdominal surgery—infection, bowel injury, hernia, and more. On top of that, a recent roundup of ADR-specific complications found that 14 percent of recipients had temporary neurological damage, and 6 percent had permanent damage. One in ten had new pain or temporary pain progression, and 18.5 percent had some damage to the involuntary nervous system.[v] That's a list that gives me pause, although the overall complication rates for ADR aren't markedly different from the complication rates for other anterior spinal fusion surgery.

My biggest concern is that those two complication rates aren't comparable. We've been performing spinal fusions in this country for fifty years, and we've seen just about every imaginable complication. There are also many, many surgeons out there with a great deal of fusion experience under their belts. With ADR, even the most experienced surgeons are new at it, and there's a higher probability that something will go wrong simply because doctors are still working out the kinks. One long-term concern relates to microscopic particle wear from the plastic insert. A similar complication has been known to occur with some types of total hip replacement surgery.

A group from the Netherlands (where they have been doing disc replacement for some time) reported on their complications from ADR. It's a very limited study; three doctors published a study of twenty-seven patients who received a brand of disc called Charité and suffered serious problems.[vi] Because the report only looked at patients with complications, and didn't include the patients without complications, it is scary. The point of the study, though, is not to figure out what percent of patients have complications, but to explore the nature of those complications.

Here's what they found:

14 patients had problems with adjacent vertebrae

4 had abdominal wall hematoma

2 men had erectile problems

16 had subsidence of the disc (it sinks into the surrounding bone)

4 patients had to have the discs removed

11 patients needed follow-up "salvage" surgery

There were also other problems, but those were the major ones. (They add up to more than twenty-seven because many patients had more than one complication.) I think that the two most important items on that list are problems with adjacent vertebrae and the need for salvage surgery. The adjacent vertebrae problems are troubling because the Charité's maker specifically claims that one of the advantages that ADR has over fusion is a decreased, or perhaps even eliminated, risk of adjacent level disease, yet here we see fourteen patients with that problem. I'm particularly concerned about it because it makes me suspicious of ADR's other claim, that it preserves motion. Although there are several possible explanations for failure of adjacent vertebrae, one of the most obvious would be that motion isn't being preserved, and that the vertebrae above and below are being stressed. We'll need more information before we can say for sure.

Salvage surgery may be an even more important issue because it's a life-threatening procedure. The artificial disc is implanted with anterior surgery (through your front). It has to be taken out the same way, and repeat anterior spine surgery is dangerous. The risk of damage to internal organs or crucial blood vessels is so high that many surgeons simply won't do repeat anterior spine procedures. Most revision surgery is done from the back and leaves the implant in place. If an artificial disc needs to be removed, though, the surgeon has no choice but to go get it from the front.

Aside from the published complications, there have been cases of the disc slipping out of place, and discs that were misaligned. This is based on only a couple years' worth of data for a device that's supposed to last a lifetime. There may be other complications that surface as more patients have the disc for more time.

The FDA acknowledges the risk of serious complications for the disc. One of their requirements for doctors who do ADR is that they also be capable of doing spinal fusion, the fallback surgery for disc replacements that fail. Although most surgeons only began doing ADR in January 2005, some patients are already getting a second surgery for a failed ADR.[vii] Upwards of 24 percent in one series required a reoperation.[viii]

One particularly thorough survey of all available research on ADR concluded: "The theoretical advantages are unproven clinically . . . early results are satisfactory. . . . Long-term results are unavailable and failure modes are unknown."[ix] It's only when there's been enough time for things to go wrong—and that could be years or decades—that the more accurate results come to the surface.

CASE STUDY

GEORGE is a forty-something accountant with back pain. Serious back pain. He went to see a surgeon, who did an MRI, and found not one but two suspect discs. He recommended disc replacement. "We're not sure which one it is," he told the unwitting George, "so we're going to do both." This didn't sound quite right to George, so he asked his primary care physician to recommend a doctor for a second opinion. He came to see me, and I told him that, under the very best of circumstances, I would only consider replacing one disc. I also told him that I didn't think he had an adequate workup. He hadn't had a CT scan or diagnostic injections, so we didn't know if he had facet joint involvement. More important, he also hadn't tried any of the alternative treatments. I didn't think he was anywhere close to considering ADR, so I sent him to a physiatrist. George is now trying nonsurgical approaches to pain management.

TOTAL DISC REPLACEMENT RESEARCH SUMMARY
- Early results of ADR are better than fusion at fixing low back pain.
- At two years, results of ADR are similar to fusion for back pain.
- ADR has a similar rate of complications to other anterior spine surgery.
- Long-term problems with disc replacement are not known.
- Up to a quarter of disc replacement patients may need follow-up surgery.
- The vast majority of patients have some condition that rules out ADR.

THE BOTTOM LINE

Because, up until now, spinal fusion has been the procedure of choice to treat low back pain, I explain in detail the problems of fixing back pain with surgery in chapter 13. Much of what I said in that chapter goes for ADR as well. As with fusion, there's the problem of pegging pain to a specific disc. As with fusion, even certainty that a particular disc is responsible doesn't guarantee results. As with fusion, many patients get worse instead of better. And, as with fusion, there is a very significant risk of complications. Unlike fusion, though, ADR hasn't been around long enough for us to fully understand what those complications are.

Some of the advantages of disc replacement are fulfilling their promise. Patients get out of the hospital earlier than they would if they'd undergone spinal fusion. They also return to activity sooner, and don't have to wear a brace. Early indications are that motion is preserved, though that may not last a lifetime. Any time a surgeon changes the structure of your bones, either by cracking or scraping or implanting a foreign object, new bone will form around the site. If enough new bone forms around an artificial disc, the mobility advantage may very well disappear.

One thing to keep in mind about ADR is that it only switches out the disc; it won't affect any other part of your spine that may be causing problems. A case in point is facet joints. Each vertebra connects to the one above it or below it in three places: the disc itself and each of the two facets, which form a kind of tripod. If those facet joints are involved in your pain at all, ADR won't fix that pain and might very well make it worse. And if your facet joints are at all arthritic, disturbing them to insert the disc is very dangerous; your spine is unlikely to settle back to a stable configuration.

All in all, the early research, the risk of complications, and the procedure's limitations leave me unwilling to perform the surgery myself, and I can't wholeheartedly recommend it for anyone. There are, however, a select few patients in very specific circumstances for whom I wouldn't absolutely rule it out.

If you think that list excludes a lot of people, you're right. One study that looked at a group of patients who'd already had fusion surgery found that fully 95 percent of them would have been disqualified for disc replacement for one reason or another.[x] If you're among the remaining 5 percent who meet all these criteria, the advantages of ADR—less invasive surgery, earlier return to activity, no brace—may make it worth the risks. Make sure, though, that you really are in that 5 percent.

If, after reading this, you think you might be one of those few, here's a list of criteria you need to meet:

- You've had disabling back pain for at least six months (try to wait longer).
- The vast majority of your pain is in your back and buttock.
- You don't have sciatica.
- Your pain is attributable to only one disc at L4-L5 or L5-S1.
- Your facet joints are not involved in your back pain, and you've had lidocaine injections to prove it.
- You've tried many other avenues, including most or all of the following: physical therapy, injections (including facet joint injections), medication, pain management, acupuncture, and chiropractic treatment.
- Your doctor has excluded other mechanical sources of pain,

including tumor, fracture, infection, spondylolisthesis, and spondylolysis.

- You don't take any medication that might affect your bones, such as prednisone.
- You don't have any of the following conditions, which may exclude you from consideration for disc replacement:

  osteoporosis

  rheumatoid arthritis (or any inflammatory arthritic condition)

  active or chronic infection

  allergy to any of the disc components
- You haven't had certain types of prior spinal surgery.

Although there are many, many patients who don't meet the criteria for ADR, there are undeniably some who do. If you're one of them, and you're considering undergoing the procedure, you should find the doctor near you who has the most experience with ADR. Remember that the longer you wait, the more experience your doctor will have and the more information we'll have about the procedure in general. Your chances of success might be that much better next month, or next year.

RED FLAGS

If any of these are true, do not proceed with total disc replacement:

- Your pain is tolerable.
- You have one of the contraindications listed above.
- You haven't tried alternative treatments.
- You're convinced it's a good idea because someone you know had it and it was successful.
- You haven't read this chapter very, very carefully.

I will add a caveat to what is generally a downbeat assessment of artificial disc replacement. As a spine surgeon, I want to see my field improve. When improvements are first introduced, they're often imperfect. Sometimes, a surgical technique that turns out to be very valuable begins its life as a spectacular failure, and I'm not writing off artificial discs altogether. I think it's possible they may be improved to the point where they perform better than conventional surgery, and I'll be keeping close tabs on the field.

In the meantime, though, there are too many unanswered questions. We don't know which disc abnormalities are the best candidates for ADR. We don't know if we can replace more than one disc. We don't know how long the discs will last. We don't know how discs will perform in patients who develop osteoporosis or arthritis. For the vast majority of patients, my advice is to wait and see.

ENDNOTES

i S. D. Boden, et al., "An AOA Critical Issue. Disc Replacements: This Time Will We Really Cure Low-Back and Neck Pain?," *Journal of Bone and Joint Surgery (Am.)* 86-A, no. 2 (2004), pp. 411–22.

ii P. C. McAfee, et al., "SB Charité Disc Replacement: Report of 60 Prospective Randomized Cases in a US Center," *Journal of Spinal Disorders & Techniques* 16 (2003), pp. 424–33.

iii R. D. Guyer, et al., "Prospective Randomized Study of the Charité Artificial Disc: Data from Two Investigational Centers," *The Spine Journal* 4, no. 6S (2004), pp. 252S–59S.

iv P. Gillet, "The Fate of the Adjacent Motion Segments."

v R. D. Guyer, D. D. Ohnmeiss, "Intervertebral Disc Prostheses," *Spine* 28, no. 15S (2003), pp. S15–S23.

vi A. van Ooij, F. C. Oner, A. J. Verbout, "Complications of Artificial Disc Replacement. A Report of 27 Patients with the SB Charité Disc," *Journal of Spinal Disorders & Techniques* 16 (2003), pp. 369–83.

vii Ibid.

viii W. S. Zeegers, et al., "Artificial Disc Replacement with the Modular Type SB Charité III: 2-Year Results in 50 Prospectively Studied Patients," *European Spine Journal* 8, no. 3 (1999), pp. 210–17.

ix P. A. Anderson, J. P. Rouleau, "Intervertebral Disc Arthroplasty," *Spine* 29, no. 23 (2004), pp. 2779–86.

x R. C. Huang, et al., "The Prevalence of Contraindications to Total Disc Replacement in a Cohort of Lumbar Surgical Patients," *Spine* 29, no. 22 (2004), pp. 2538–41.

Chapter 16

MINIMALLY INVASIVE TECHNIQUES

When it comes to incisions, size matters. Gaping holes require more time to heal and open the door to risk of infection, muscle damage, scar tissue, and bleeding. That's why, in just about all kinds of surgery, there is a trend toward high-tech equipment that makes surgery possible with smaller incisions and, consequently, less hospital time, less recovery time, and a reduced risk of complications. Spine surgery is no exception. There are new devices and techniques that both change how traditional procedures are done and enable new procedures.

If you're thinking about getting a minimally invasive procedure done, you have to keep in mind that "minimally invasive" doesn't mean "effective." It just means minimally invasive. And while that's generally a good thing, it doesn't mean that you should consider the surgery any less carefully than you would a maximally invasive procedure.

Smaller incisions are good, and some procedures get better results when they're performed with minimally invasive techniques. Other procedures, though, are actually more dangerous, and have poorer results. Partly, that's because some of these techniques are on the steep end of the learning curve and we haven't yet learned when they're likely to be most effective. They're also often harder to do than traditional surgery; you have to work very precisely, with equipment that takes a while to get familiar with.

So don't be seduced by high-tech gadgetry. If you're considering one of these procedures, evaluate it on its merits.

ELECTROTHERMAL AND RADIOFREQUENCY DISC TREATMENTS

These are procedures that go out on a limb. They're used only to treat discogenic pain—not herniated discs, not stenosis, not bone spurs. The theory is that if a particular disc is causing pain, you can stop the pain by destroying the painful part of the disc. The firm, outer part of the disc—the annulus—is believed to be the painful part because it's the only part that has nerves in it. If the nerves die, so will the pain. Again, that's the theory.

The agent of destruction is energy—heat, cold, laser, radiofrequency—which, when applied directly to a disc, kills those nerves. It also changes the structure of collagen, and eliminates inflammatory chemicals, although the degree to which those factors enter into the pain-stopping equation is questionable. Once those things are all gone, though, your pain should stop. In theory.

If you're thinking about one of these procedures, you should keep in mind that we don't really know what makes a disc painful. Given all of that uncertainty, it shouldn't surprise you that we don't really know whether we can neutralize a painful disc by zapping it with energy.

Let's get away from the theory for a minute and get to the practice. Here's how the procedure goes. You get a shot of local anesthetic in your back, and your surgeon inserts a catheter into your spine. He uses a fluoroscope to watch the progress of the catheter as he guides it to the suspect disc. Then he inserts an electrode through the catheter into the disc, and zaps it with some kind of energy that kills the nerves in the outer part of the disc. Two hours later, you should be able to get up and go home.

This kind of procedure goes by many names, including:

intradiscal electrothermal therapy (IDET)
intradiscal electrothermal annuloplasty (IEA)
intradiscal electrothermoplasty
intradiscal thermal modulation (ITM)
radiofrequency discal nucleoplasty
coblation nucleoplasty

They're coming up with names faster than you can say spondylolisthesis, so it's not useful to analyze these one by one. They're all similar; they just use different forms of energy to do the zapping. Some use thermal energy (heat). Some use radio waves (which also produce heat). Some use lasers (in a procedure that is also occasionally used for herniated discs rather than discogenic pain, and I've broken out that function below). Some use cold (cryoablation). You don't have to remember them all. You only have to remember that no one form of energy seems to work better than any other. They're all equally ineffective.

In 2005, researchers in Australia published a randomized, double-blind, controlled study (that's the best kind) of IDET versus placebo surgery. The good news that came out of that study is that IDETs seem safe; there were no significant complications. The bad news is that they didn't relieve pain any better than a placebo.[i]

In general, at least half of the patients who undergo electrothermal procedures see no improvement. In the best of hands, and under the most stringent selection criteria, about four in ten see some improvement.[ii] And not all studies reported results that good. In one study, 97 percent of patients still had back pain, and an unfortunate 58 percent reported the same or more pain after being zapped.[iii] Looking at all the research, I have to conclude that there is no good evidence that this procedure works. In doing so, I'm in good company; many doctors question its basic premise.[iv]

Beyond its not working, though, is the risk that it will make things worse. The possibility of more pain is the obvious downside to these procedures, but there's also a less obvious one. We don't know the long-term consequences of killing the nerves in a disc, or of changing its chemical structure. Could it lead to premature degeneration, which could in turn lead to more pain down the road, or even the necessity for more serious surgery? The same study that reported that 97 percent of subjects still had pain also found that 30 percent of patients needed major reconstructive spine surgery within two years of having the procedure done. Although we can't specifically blame the procedure for the need for surgery, it's not a good sign. We don't have a good sense of the real long-term risk of having a procedure like this done, but we do know that zapping the disc does permanent damage to proteins and collagen, vital parts of a functional disc. It may also affect the water content, and since water is part of what keeps a disc soft enough to absorb shock, that may have adverse long-term consequences. How adverse? How long? We just don't know, but the uncertainty itself is a risk that you should take into account if you're considering one of these procedures.

Although the risk of complications from the procedures themselves is small, it exists. There have been reports of nerve injuries, infections, and damage from broken catheters.

Now that I've told you I don't believe that these procedures alleviate pain, and I've alerted you to the possibility of adverse long- and short-term consequences, I'm going to point out that these procedures are still a lot safer than fusion surgery. If you're on the verge of fusion, and your doctor recommends one of these procedures as a last-ditch attempt to stop your pain, it's hard for me to tell you unequivocally not to do it. If the alternative really is fusion, you don't have much to lose.

PERCUTANEOUS ENDOSCOPIC LASER DISCECTOMY (PELD)

You read about microdiscectomy—the procedure by which the herniated part of a disc is removed—in chapter 12. An endoscopic discectomy is a procedure that accomplishes the same goal, but with special tools that enable the surgeon to work through a smaller incision. The primary tool is an endoscope, a long, thin tube with a microscope on the end, which lets your surgeon see the herniated disc without looking at it directly. It's kind of like a periscope on a submarine, only the endoscope also magnifies the image.

Once the endoscope is in place, your surgeon will insert the laser. Instead of physically scraping off the herniation, the laser denatures and vaporizes the tissue behind the herniated disc. If you're wondering exactly how denaturation and vaporization of tissue behind the disc removes your herniated disc, I'm with you. I don't know. There is very little research in the area.

There is also not much research data on the effectiveness of PELD. What we do know is that it's very demanding; it requires practice and precision, and the cost of a mistake could be severely damaged nerves. Don't be seduced by the "laser" in the title. This procedure is no safer than a conventional laminectomy, and there's no evidence that it's more effective. I don't recommend this procedure.

ENDOSCOPIC DISCECTOMY

This is another version of a minimally invasive discectomy. It differs from the laser procedure in that the surgeon uses more conventional means to scrape off the herniated portion of the disc.

This procedure sounds very good in theory, but it has a couple of problems in practice. The first is one that patients are unlikely to think about: it's technically demanding and theoretically more dangerous than a standard discectomy. It takes a lot of practice to maneuver a tiny tube in a small space, and to work with an indirect view of what you're supposed to be removing. It takes time to master the procedure, which is one reason that endoscopic discectomies haven't really caught on.

The second problem is that the tools aren't good enough. Unlike in other endoscopic procedures, an endoscope for discectomy doesn't give me the view, the access, or the maneuverability that I get with a traditional microdiscectomy. As the tools are refined and improved, I hope that the procedure will get easier, more effective, and more common. That doesn't help you if you're thinking about surgery right now, though. If that's the case, the question is whether endoscopic discectomies work better than other kinds of discectomies right now. The answer is that we don't have enough data to say for sure.

The incision for a standard discectomy is not very big (usually about an inch or so). The advantage of endoscopic discectomy for a couple of smaller incisions does not seem to balance out the dangers involved. As of now, I do not perform endoscopic discectomies, and I do not recommend them.

FACET NEUROTOMY

A neurotomy is the cutting of a nerve, and in this case it's the nerve that carries the sensation from a painful facet joint.

Arthritis can cause degeneration of the cartilage of the facet joint, which is one of the places where two adjacent vertebrae meet. If the degeneration is severe, the joint can become painful in the same way that a knee or hip with worn cartilage can.

When pain is thought to come from a facet joint, it's called facet syndrome. And, just as you feel pain from a degenerated joint in the knee itself, pain from a facet joint is back pain. If most of your pain is radicular (felt in the leg), it's unlikely that facet syndrome is the problem, and therefore unlikely that a neurotomy will help you.

A neurotomy doesn't fix your facet joint; it just severs the conduit by which the sensation of pain is passed to the brain. The theory (and there are a lot of theories in this chapter) is that, without the conduit, you won't get the sensation. Since there's no way to repair the facet joint, cutting off communication is the only way to keep the pain from reaching your brain. Those communications are cut when the nerve is severed, which can be done either by physically cutting through it or by cauterizing it with energy of some kind. Whatever the method, the goal is the same: block the pain.

The actual procedure is done in much the same way that the electrothermal procedures in the section above are done. A catheter is inserted through the skin in the back, and an electrode goes in through the catheter. The surgeon watches with a fluoroscope, and then zaps the nerve when the electrode is in place.

If it's certain that your facet joint is causing pain, this procedure might help you. One clue as to whether it will or won't help you is a diagnostic facet block (see page 176). The facet block numbs the nerve or the joint, and if that makes you feel better, it's a pretty safe bet that you've found the source of your pain. In that case, a neurotomy may ease your pain, at least in the short term. If the facet block doesn't work, it's likely that the neurotomy won't either. Although the facet block isn't a sure indicator, I recommend that you have it before a neurotomy. It doesn't have to be a separate procedure—your doctor can do it just before the neurotomy, using the same catheter—so it doesn't add any risk.

There's no good, thorough research on neurotomies, but there is some limited evidence that they can help a very small, specific group of patients whose pain is definitely established to originate in the facet joint.[iv] If that's you, a neurotomy may be worth trying.

VERTEBROPLASTY AND KYPHOPLASTY

I'm grouping these two procedures together because they're similar in concept and they treat the same condition—compression fractures. Here's the basic idea. When a vertebra collapses, the outer shell (the hard cortical bone) falls in on the soft core (the marrow). It will almost always heal itself, but it takes time, it restricts motion, and it can be painful. Vertebroplasty and kyphoplasty facilitate the healing by filling the vertebra with liquid bone cement, which, as it hardens, stabilizes the vertebra.

Both procedures use a small tube with a tiny device like a caulking gun. The surgeon maneuvers the tube (using a fluoroscope) into the fractured vertebra and injects the bone cement. The key difference between the two procedures is that in vertebroplasty, the cement is injected directly into the vertebra; in kyphoplasty, the surgeon first passes a balloon into the vertebra, inflates it to make a cavity, removes the balloon, and fills the cavity with the cement.

Kyphoplasty claims two advantages over vertebroplasty. The first is that it can restore some height and alignment (two of the problems with compression fractures, described on page 60). The balloon restores some of the vertebra's pre-fracture shape, and then the cement holds it there. This sure sounds good, but, so far, we don't have any data on whether it matters in the long run. We know that lots of patients do very well with vertebrae that heal in their collapsed shape, and we can't say for sure that restoring (or, more likely, partly restoring) the shape of the vertebra improves outcomes.

The second advantage is reduced risks of bone cement leaks. Leakage is a problem with both procedures, but the cavity created by the balloon used in kyphoplasty may help contain the cement. Also, with vertebroplasty the cement is injected under pressure, and so it may be more likely to leak outside the bone. That might or might not be a problem, depending on where the leak is. The bone cement itself isn't toxic, but it could end up in the spinal canal and compress nerves, or get into the blood system, raising the possibility of a lung embolism (which is very rare but can be deadly). Some reports indicate bone cement with vertebroplasty leaks out of the bone up to 48 percent of the time, even though complications are rarely reported.[v] Kyphoplasty is newer, and so there's not a lot of information on complication rates.

Kyphoplasty has one disadvantage: it's harder for the surgeon to do. It's more complicated, it's technically demanding, and it takes a little longer. Both vertebroplasty and kyphoplasty, though, are safe, effective procedures. There aren't many complications other than the chance of leakage. As with any surgery, there's the chance of infection and surgeon error. Some doctors prefer to do the procedures with general anesthesia, and then the risks of anesthesia need to be considered, but I prefer to do them with only mild sedation, so my patients avoid the risk of anesthesia.

There are some conditions that can make either of these procedures ill-advised. If you have an infection, a bleeding disorder, or an allergy to any of the medications used, you need to consult carefully with your doctor. Most of my fracture patients, though, aren't in any of these categories, and I do many of these procedures (primarily kyphoplasty). My patients are generally up and walking hours after the procedure, and experience significant pain relief. Patients who get a second fracture elsewhere after having had a kyphoplasty almost invariably ask me to treat their second fracture the same way.

So far, there aren't any head-to-head comparison trials of the two procedures (although they're in progress). I think they are both useful, safe, and generally successful. There aren't many procedures in this book that I recommend as enthusiastically as I can recommend vertebroplasty and kyphoplasty for compression fractures.

ENDNOTES

i B. J. Freeman, et al., "A Randomized, Double-Blind, Controlled Trial: Intradiscal Electrothermal Therapy *Versus* Placebo for the Treatment of Chronic Discogenic Low Back Pain," *Spine* 30, no. 21 (2005), pp. 2369–77.

ii K. J. Pauza, et al., "A Randomized, Placebo-controlled Trial of Intradiscal Electrothermal Therapy for the Treatment of Discogenic Low Back Pain," *The Spine Journal* 4 (2004), pp. 27–35.

iii T. T. Davis, et al., "The IDET Procedure for Chronic Discogenic Low Back Pain," *Spine* 29, no. 7 (2004), pp. 752–56.

iv C. W. Slipman, et al., "A Critical Review of the Evidence for the Use of Zygapophysial Injections and Radiofrequency Denervation in the Treatment of Low Back Pain," *The Spine Journal* 3 (2003), pp. 310–16.

v A. Pérez-Higueras, et al. "Percutaneous Vertebroplasty: Long-term Clinical and Radiological Outcome," *Neuroradiology* 44 (2002), pp. 950–54.

AFTER THE SURGERY

Care and Complications

Chapter 17

GENERAL COMPLICATIONS

In my experience, the biggest fear of a patient undergoing spine surgery is waking up paralyzed. And with good reason; it's the next-to-worst-case scenario. While paralysis is a real risk, it's a small one. There are other, more likely but less serious complications that every patient needs to understand and consider. For every instance of paralysis, there are hundreds of infections, leaks of spinal fluid, blood clots, and blood vessel damage.

I don't mean to scare you. Well, actually, I guess I do mean to scare you—at least a little. In my experience, patients downplay the possibility of complications. They believe that the probability is remote, and that it won't happen to them. And it is true that the probability of most of the complications in this chapter *is* remote, but any surgical procedure puts you at risk for one or more of them, so the chance of experiencing at least one may not be as small as you think. Besides, a small chance is cold comfort when you *do* have the problem.

The risks vary widely. Simple procedures, like kyphoplasty, have fewer, smaller risks. Complicated procedures, like multilevel fusion, have more, bigger risks. This chapter is a rundown of the most common, including their likelihood, as well as guidance on how to prevent them and what to do about them if they happen to you. I've included risks that are specific to, or particularly common with, spine surgery. But remember that all surgery has some risks, including infection, hematoma, blood clots, retained foreign bodies (the clamp left in your abdomen), urinary tract problems, and anesthesia risks, and you need to consider these as well, even though I don't cover them in this book.

DURING SURGERY

Paralysis and nerve injury are the scariest complications, and the ones that patients are most worried about. The damage from nerve injury can be major or minor, with paralysis being the most serious consequence. Any nerve injury, though, even if it only causes some minor numbness and tingling, can have long-term consequences. And, although the incidence of nerve injury during surgery is small, it's large enough to be the cause of legitimate concern.

Nerves are like the electrical lines in your house. You've got one central hookup to the utility company, and then branches leading to all your rooms. With nerves, the central hookup is the spinal column, which leads directly to the brain (the utility company, if I'm not stretching this analogy too far). The branches go to your limbs, organs, muscles, joints, skin, and just about everywhere else. From there, they carry signals to your brain (you're hungry, you stubbed your toe, it's cold out, your hair's on fire). Your brain sends signals back (eat, yell, shiver, douse). Without nerves, you're completely cut off.

During surgery, nerves are at risk. Your surgeon is using sharp tools, and the nerves are right there. Besides getting cut, nerves can also be stretched or compressed when your surgeon has to move them to reach an area they're blocking. Symptoms of nerve damage include weakness in your legs, numbness, tingling, pain, feelings of heightened sensation, loss of bowel or bladder function, and impaired sexual function. If your nerves are stretched or compressed, the injury may be temporary. If the nerve is cut, the ends can be sewn together, but there is little chance you'll recover the function.

Usually, the treatment for nerve damage is to wait. In most cases, your symptoms will either improve or they won't, and nothing can change that. There are cases when something—an implant, a hematoma, or an infection—is pressing on the nerve, causing the symptoms, and it can be removed. Those cases excepted, the nerves are left to heal themselves.

There is one specific kind of nerve injury that my male patients are particularly concerned about: retrograde ejaculation. This can happen when nerves controlling one of the sphincter muscles to the bladder are damaged. When that happens, sperm is ejaculated into the bladder rather than out of the penis. This is only a risk in anterior lumbar surgery, and the risk is much higher if your surgeon goes straight through the abdominal cavity (transperitoneal) than it is if he goes around your abdominal cavity (retroperitoneal).[i] Estimates for this risk vary from under 1 percent to over 5 percent.[ii] If you are male and you might want to have children after an anterior surgery, talk to your doctor about preoperative sperm banking.

There is also a remote chance of nerve injury following any surgical procedure. A slipped implant, a hematoma, or an infection can put pressure on the spinal nerves. A particularly dangerous form of this is postsurgical cauda equina syndrome. You know all about cauda equina syndrome from chapter 5, and the postsurgical variety is one of the most dangerous complications of spine surgery. Fortunately, it's also rare. The first symptom of postsurgical cauda equina syndrome is often either incontinence or urinary retention. Because these are also very common side effects of anesthesia and narcotic pain relievers, it's easy to miss the early stages. If you have either of these symptoms, or any new neurological symptom in the postoperative period, alert your doctor immediately.

Wrong site surgery is exactly what it sounds like. Your doctor operates on the wrong part of your spine. Although this can happen with any kind of surgery, when spines are involved there are a lot of identical structures in very close proximity. Even so, it doesn't happen often, and it's happening less and less since there's been a national initiative to address the problem. You can help avoid it by double-checking with everyone concerned with your surgery that your herniated disc is L4-L5, not L3-L4. Let that be the last thing you talk to your surgeon and nursing staff about as you're wheeled into the operating room. As silly as it sounds, it's not unreasonable to ask your surgeon to write it on your back in indelible ink before you go into the operating room. Make sure the site of surgery is clearly stated on the informed consent form you sign before the surgery. The best strategy for wrong site surgery is to do everything you can to prevent it.

Spinal fluid leak is when cerebrospinal fluid (CSF), which is supposed to be contained by a lining around your nerves called the dura, escapes. (Some surgical procedures, although none we cover in this book, require that the dura be entered in order to get to the nerves.) Although surgeons try not to let accidental dural tears happen, it is sometimes very difficult to avoid. The risk is higher with older patients, who have thinner dura, and in reoperation surgery, where scar tissue makes avoiding dural leaks more difficult. Leaks are much more likely in some procedures than in others, and your doctor can tell you ahead of time whether your risk is high or low.

The key to managing it is to keep the leakage to a minimum. If the leak is sealed and only a small amount of fluid gets out, it's generally harmless. If, however, the fluid continues to leak after surgery, something has to be done. Normally, the central nervous system is completely contained, and closed up from the rest of your body, so it's at minimal risk for things like infection. When you have a spinal fluid leak, it opens your nervous system up to the outside world.

Luckily, the fix for spinal fluid leaks is relatively easy. Most of them are caught and repaired in the operating room. Sometimes that repair is insufficient and you'll need additional treatment post-op. Often, that's just a couple of days of bed rest or a special drain. If the leak is severe and persistent (which is unusual), you may need follow-up surgery to close the leak.

Injuries to veins and arteries happen during surgery. Always. You can't have any surgical procedure without some blood loss. Most of the vessels cut during spine surgery are small veins and arteries, similar to the kind you injure with a paper cut. Bones also bleed (orthopedic surgeons have no idea where the expression "bone-dry" comes from), and the more bone is cut, the greater the blood loss.

Anterior fusion has a higher risk of blood vessel damage than any other procedure I talk about in this book, for the simple reason that the doctor has to go through the front, and move very large blood vessels out of the way. The aorta and vena cava run down the front of the spine, and each splits at about the L4-L5 level, making surgery on that site riskier than other levels.

If you lose enough blood on the table, you may require a transfusion. In general, that need shouldn't arise for a simple procedure like a laminectomy. If you're planning to have a more complex procedure, which lasts longer and cuts into more structures, you may want to plan for the possibility of a transfusion. Talk to your doctor about whether you want to give blood ahead of time just in case.

AFTER SURGERY

Bedsores can happen after any surgery, but I'm including them because there's still a widespread idea that bed rest is the way to recover from spine surgery. It absolutely is not, and bedsores are just one of the reasons. They don't sound so bad—we've all had sores, right?—but they can be very dangerous. They develop where there is consistent pressure on the skin (their other name is pressure sores) for a long enough time that a wound develops. One of the reasons they're dangerous is that the sores may not show until days after the damage has occurred, and so the deterioration is significant before treatment begins. Sores can hurt, they can get infected, and they can take months to heal.

Treatment is generally avoiding pressure on the sore, often supplemented by careful and regular wound cleaning. If the sore is very bad, it may need to be cleaned surgically.

The optimal treatment, though, is prevention. The best thing you can do after surgery—to prevent bedsores, to facilitate healing, and to get back to your life—is to be up and about as soon as possible. When you absolutely, positively have to be in bed (and you will have to be, for a short time), make sure that you turn frequently. If you can't turn yourself, get help. And pay particular attention to the tailbone and heels, which are some of the sites most susceptible to bedsores.

FAILED BACK SURGERY SYNDROME (FBSS)

Sounds horrible, doesn't it? It is. FBSS encompasses anything that happens to you after surgery that doesn't fall into another category. It is characterized by pain that no one knows the source of. It could be a painful disc, it could be pseudarthrosis, or it could be damaged facets. The blame is often laid at the feet of damaged muscles. When fusion is done through the back, there's a chance that the lumbar back muscles can be affected. This may happen because the nerve conduits to the muscle can be disrupted. No one knows why it happens, but it results in the muscles disengaging from the rest of your nervous system, and they atrophy.

Another possible cause of FBSS is arachnoiditis, an inflammation of the lining of the nerves that is a rare complication of a laminectomy. The lining, called the arachnoid (presumably because it looks like a spider's web), is just inside the dura. If it gets inflamed, it can cause nerve-related pain that is very difficult to treat. One treatment option being offered for FBSS (and some other chronic pain conditions) is a spinal cord stimulator, a surgically implanted device designed to manage pain by stimulating the spinal cord with very low-level electrical impulses. Not much is known about the safety and efficacy of these devices but, as an option of last resort, if your pain is not responsive to other treatments, a stimulator may be worth considering.

FBSS causes pain and loss of function. We don't know how often it happens and we don't know what causes it, but it's often implicated when people have pain that can't otherwise be explained. It is a difficult situation for any patient to deal with. Most of the time there isn't a surgical solution; a multidisciplinary approach to the problem is needed, including psychological support, physical rehabilitation, medication, and pain management.

CASE STUDY

JOAN is single mom in her thirties who worked as a secretary. She had sciatica from a herniated disc that hadn't responded to nonsurgical alternatives. Her surgeon did a laminectomy, which should have solved the problem. It didn't. During the procedure, there was a spinal fluid leak. A serious infection followed and Joan ended up undergoing two additional surgeries to fix the leak and clear out the infection. After all that was done, she came to see me for a second opinion because she still had the original sciatica, and now had significant back pain. At that point, her only possible alternative was major reconstructive surgery, a procedure I thought she was too beaten down, both emotionally and physically, to endure. I advised her to consider reconstruction once she felt a little stronger and more emotionally stable.

SUMMARY

The likelihood of some of the more serious complications is slim. But, if a complication happens to you, it can be serious, even life-threatening. When a complication occurs, patients react in different ways. Some get angry, others get frustrated, and many become fearful. These reactions are all normal. Managing these feelings is part of the process of healing. Often patients benefit from counseling or support groups.

I want to point out, though, that every surgeon who does enough of this surgery has patients with complications. I feel that what separates one surgeon from another is how he manages them. You should expect your surgeon to recognize a complication as soon as possible, tell you about it candidly, and treat it appropriately. He should explain clearly what happened, talk about why it might have happened, and lay out what, if any, options there are for further treatment. Above all, your surgeon should be accessible and communicative.

When I have a patient who suffers a complication, I work openly and thoroughly with my patient to do everything possible to right the situation. Complications are a fact of surgery. Poorly handled complications don't have to be.

ENDNOTE

i R. C. Sasso, J. K. Burkus, J. LeHuec, "Retrograde Ejaculation After Anterior Lumbar Interbody Fusion," *Spine* 28, no. 10 (2003), pp. 1023–26.

ii J. C. Flynn, C. T. Price, "Sexual Complications of Anterior Fusion of the Lumbar Spine," *Spine* 9, no. 9 (1984), pp. 489–92.

   H. Tiusanen, et al., "Retrograde Ejaculation After Anterior Interbody Lumbar Fusion," *European Spine Journal* 4 (1995), pp. 339–42.

Chapter 18

REVISION SURGERY

The one thing you should be sure of by the time you get to this chapter is that spinal surgery doesn't always work out the way you'd hope. Not even surgery with a good track record for a specific diagnosis is foolproof. Whether it's because a procedure doesn't fix the problem, or something goes wrong in the operating room, or the problem is fixed but recurs, some patients who opt for surgery end up having to opt for it again.

Lots of things are easier the second time around, but spine surgery isn't one of them. The very fact that your back has been operated on once already makes the second procedure more difficult and riskier. There may be scar tissue that encases nerves and makes them harder to find and to move. There may be bone removed that makes the removal of more bone a risk for instability. There may be broken hardware that has done more damage to a site than was there in the first place. Although the procedures for revision surgery are often the same as for the original surgery, I've put them in a separate chapter because the considerations and complications are a little different the second time.

Another reason revision surgery is different is that you might very well be upset. If you think you need a revision because your surgeon made a mistake during the original procedure or recommended the wrong surgery in the first place, it's perfectly natural to be frustrated. I don't blame you, and chances are your doctor doesn't either. But anger can make an already difficult process worse, and the best thing you can do is try to understand why the repeat surgery is necessary and focus on fixing the problem.

The need for revision surgery may arise anytime after the initial surgery, from the next day to decades later. If you develop a hematoma (a collection of blood) in a place where it presses on a nerve, you may need an emergency procedure to evacuate it. If an infection develops, the wound may need a surgical cleaning called an irrigation and debridement (I&D). Because all of these are risks of surgery in general, I'm not going to cover them. I just want you to be aware that they exist.

Most causes of spine-specific revision surgery fall into one of five categories:

revision laminectomy
    recurrent herniated disc
    recurrent spinal stenosis
hardware failure
fusion non-union
adjacent level disease
postoperative instability

REVISION LAMINECTOMY

Fortunately, second-time procedures aren't always necessary for recurrent stenosis or disc reherniation. If conservative treatments, such as medication and physical therapy, didn't work for your first problem, that doesn't mean they won't work for your second. I know it's demoralizing to go back to square one and try the nonsurgical approaches all over again, but that's preferable to the alternative.

Revision laminectomy for a herniated disc: A first-time laminectomy to relieve pressure on a nerve from a herniated disc is a straightforward procedure (described in excruciating detail in chapter 12). If the condition recurs, the fix is the same. The chance that you'll need that fix, though, may be higher than you think. Estimates vary from study to study, country to country, and population to population, but the chance of needing a second-time surgery at some point down the road for a herniated disc hovers in the 5–19 percent range.[i]

There are two issues that make a second laminectomy riskier than a first: scar tissue and instability. Let's tackle scar tissue first.

Chances are good that you're familiar with scar tissue. I'm willing to bet you've got some on your knees or your hands. The part you can see, though, is just the tip of the iceberg. Scar tissue also forms inside. After your first procedure, it's likely that scar tissue formed at the site of the incision, and not just on the skin. It also forms around the structures in the spine. The amount varies by the type of surgery and the individual patient's propensity to form scar tissue.

Scar tissue is hard and rubbery, and it often forms in such a way as to encase the nerves. Once that happens, it's harder to find the nerves, harder to move them out of the way, and easier to damage them. To make matters more complicated, scar tissue and herniated disc material look very similar on an MRI, so it's hard to tell them apart if you are having a problem after surgery. The reason that this is important is because surgery to remove scar tissue rarely helps; surgery to remove herniated disc material may help. Even when we use contrast dye to enhance the MRI, which makes the distinction more clear, it's not always obvious. (The key difference is that scar tissue has blood vessels and disc material doesn't, and if the scan sees the dye, which flows through blood vessels, then the material is probably scar tissue. Even so, it's not always possible to distinguish one from the other.)

Because scar tissue can block access to the material that has to be removed, the hole that your surgeon made in your lamina the first time around may not be big enough to work through. And that brings us to the second risk: instability.

There is a risk of instability in every laminectomy, but it's very small in a first-time laminectomy for a herniated disc. If, however, your surgeon has to enlarge the hole, or make a second hole, the risk of instability is higher. One study found that among patients getting a second laminectomy for a recurrent herniated disc, 44 percent also got fusion because the surgeon thought that enough bone was being removed that they were at risk for instability.[ii] I'm citing this study because it's one of the few we have, but I don't want you to think there is a 44 percent chance you will need a fusion for this type of surgery. The fact that the surgeon did the fusion doesn't necessarily mean that a fusion was required. It just means that enough bone was removed that the surgeon was concerned about instability. I almost never recommend fusion with second-time laminectomy surgery for a herniated disc.

Besides scar tissue and instability risks, second-time laminectomies also have increased odds of spinal fluid leaks, infection, and nerve damage. There is not a lot of data on how much those odds are increased. The same study that found that 44 percent of second-time laminectomies required fusion also found a 12 percent incidence of dural tears (which cause spinal fluid leaks), but there are no good comparisons of first-time to second-time laminectomies. What I can tell you is that the risk of complications in a first-time laminectomy is very small. The risk the second time is a little higher.

If you're considering fusion for revision of a herniated disc, the primary consideration isn't instability, but rather the disc itself. If it has herniated twice, there's a chance it will continue to herniate. There is also a possibility that the reason it is herniating is that instability is causing abnormal motion at the site. In the first case, it makes sense to take the disc out of the lineup because it's causing trouble. In the second case, it makes sense to fuse the motion segment because *it's* causing trouble.

Nevertheless, I do not routinely recommend fusion for a second-time laminectomy for a herniated disc. The same study that looked at second-time complications compared success rates of a second laminectomy alone and a second laminectomy with fusion for reherniated discs, and found them to be statistically similar.[iii] By the third time around, though, I think fusions are often justifiable. The kind of fusion usually employed for revision surgery for a third herniation is a posterior procedure that combines fusion and decompression. The herniation is on the posterior side, and so it's hard to remove with an anterior procedure. That means you can have a posterolateral, TLIF-, or PLIF-type fusion (see page 219).

Sometimes doctors recommend a fusion with the second laminectomy/discectomy not for any of these reasons, but because of the presence of back pain. In my view (and all we have here are views because there's no good data) that decision should be weighed carefully with your surgeon.

Revision laminectomy for spinal stenosis: For recurrent stenosis, the issues are the same: scar tissue and instability. However, the number of patients requiring revision surgery is higher.

One study found that almost one in four stenosis patients needed revision surgery inside a decade.[iv]

For both scar tissue and instability, the issue plays an important role if your stenosis recurs at the same level as your prior surgery (see above). If, however, your condition recurs at an adjacent level of your spine, then the issues are less important.

The considerations in making the laminectomy-fusion combination decision are different for stenosis and herniated discs because the reasons a fusion might be appropriate are different. For stenosis, the issue is instability in the form of spondylolisthesis, scoliosis, or kyphosis, and the usual determinant of whether a fusion is appropriate is the amount of bone removed. If, in the surgeon's judgment, the total removed in the first and second procedures put you at risk for spondylolisthesis, scoliosis, or kyphosis, he will probably recommend a fusion. There are no guidelines for when this is the right decision, and it's purely a matter of your doctor's experience and best judgment.

If you do end up getting a second laminectomy for stenosis, your surgeon may raise the issue of doing a fusion along with it.

HARDWARE FAILURE

"Failure" covers a wide range of problems. Implants can dislodge, break, migrate, and pull out of the bone. Fortunately, failure doesn't automatically mean a second surgery. There are two reasons you may need revision surgery if your hardware fails. First, your doctor may have to retrieve failed hardware if it causes pain or threatens damage. Second, you may have to get another fusion to accomplish the goal the first one didn't accomplish because the hardware failed.

If you have a rod that broke or a screw that pulled out of a bone in your back, your instinct is probably to get it out, and I know the advice to leave it there is counterintuitive. But if it's not causing you pain, and it's not positioned in such a way that it could damage something important, leaving it there is exactly what you should do. The risks of letting it alone, which are minimal, are dwarfed by the risks of taking it out.

The larger question of hardware failure is whether it means the fusion also failed, and whether you have to do anything about that. If the hardware didn't have a chance to do its job, the best thing to do is to give it time to see if the fusion fuses anyway. If it doesn't, you're on to . . .

FUSION NON-UNION (PSEUDARTHROSIS)

This is a tricky one. As you know from chapter 13, many fusions never fuse. As you also know, it doesn't always matter. Often, a fusion that hasn't fused will have the same results as a fusion that has, which is one of the reasons I question the use of fusion in many circumstances. If, however, your fusion non-union means you're experiencing the same symptoms that drove you to surgery in the first place, you may need a revision.

To fix a non-union, your surgeon may choose to go in from a different access point. If your first procedure was an interbody fusion (where your disc was removed and replaced with a spacer), your second might be a posterior fusion (where the back side is fused), or the other way around. Either way, it brings on a different set of risks.

If the first fusion was through the front, doctors will go far out of their way not to do the second fusion that way, because the risk of damage to the blood vessels is very high, primarily because of scar tissue. I know doctors who simply won't perform that surgery. The good news is that if your doctor goes through the front the first time and the back the second time, the risks of the second procedure are about the same as the risks from a first-time posterior fusion.

If your first fusion was an ALIF, your doctor will probably do either a posterolateral or posterior fusion the second time around. He won't go so far as to replace the disc again; he'll just fuse the back, because that has a high probability of solving the problem. This surgery is always done with instrumentation, because a solid fusion was important enough to require a second procedure in the first place.

If your doctor went in from the back the first time, it's reasonable to do it that way again the second time, because any risks associated with second-time surgery at the same site may be outweighed by the risks of going through your abdomen. Whether or not your first fusion was instrumented, it's possible your second one will be. Remember that the only reason you're getting this surgery is that your fusion needed to fuse and it didn't. That means minimizing the chance for a second pseudarthrosis is a high priority.

ADJACENT LEVEL DISEASE

If you've already read the fusion chapter, then you know all about adjacent level disease (see page 230). When one level of your spine is fused, it puts additional stress on the levels above and below, which now have to move more to make up for the fact that the fused level isn't moving at all. Unlike other fusion revisions, which happen because a fusion doesn't work, revision for adjacent level disease is sometimes required because a fusion works exactly the way it's supposed to.

Adjacent level disease can happen months or decades after fusion surgery, but the considerations in deciding whether to reoperate are the same. The primary consideration is, of course, pain. If you can live with it, live with it.

Re-fusing for adjacent level disease has the same risks as refusing for other reasons (although, because the surgery is at a different level, scar tissue plays a smaller role), and one additional risk. Because you're fusing the level next to a fusion, you're going to end up with a larger immobile segment. It may be two levels instead of one, or three instead of two. That means the stress on the levels above and below that larger segment will be even greater than the stresses that made you get adjacent level disease in the first place. Besides, the fact that you've already got adjacent level disease may mean that you're susceptible to it, and will be likely to experience a domino effect, where level after level succumbs. I've seen patients who have undergone several separate surgeries, and I don't want you to be one of them. Put surgery off as long as you can, and try to find other ways to manage the pain.

Adjacent level disease has disparate causes, and, in turn, causes disparate problems. It's impossible to make a blanket recommendation about whether revision surgery is necessary, what kind of surgery that should be, or whether it should be instrumented.

POSTOPERATIVE INSTABILITY

This is a catchall category for just about anything that can go wrong with spine surgery. All of the common causes of postsurgical problems are covered in the previous categories, and the less common are lumped together here. Sometimes a surgical procedure can cause a vertebra to slip out of place. (The technical name for this is iatrogenic spondylolisthesis, which just means a slipped bone caused by your surgery.) More rarely, scoliosis or kyphosis, each an abnormal curvature, can be a result of surgery. Because the causes for postoperative instability are many and varied, it's impossible to make a general recommendation. You can find information on each of the conditions that cause it elsewhere in this book, and in the meantime the golden rule applies: If you can manage the problem without surgery, do so.

CASE STUDY

YOLANDA is a woman in her fifties who came to me two years ago with what could have been mild stenosis but what could also have just been degenerative changes in her spine. She had some pain, but no neurogenic claudication. I recommended, strongly, against surgery, but surgery was what she wanted and she found a doctor to do it. Within a year after a laminectomy, she started experiencing back pain worse than her original symptoms. She came back to me, and I found that the vertebra that had been operated on had slipped out of line. The spondylolisthesis was causing her intense low back pain, which we tried to manage without surgery, with no success. Eventually, we opted for a spinal fusion. She's doing fine, but it's quite possible she would have been fine if she hadn't had the laminectomy in the first place. It's better to be fine after no surgeries than after two.

ENDNOTES

i I. Keskimäki, et al., "Reoperations After Lumbar Disc Surgery: A Population-based Study of Regional and Interspeciality Variations," *Spine* 25, no. 12 (2000), pp. 1500–8.

ii T. Fu, et al., "Long-term Results of Disc Excision for Recurrent Lumbar Disc Herniation with or Without Posterolateral Fusion," *Spine* 30, no. 24 (2005), pp. 2830–34.

iii Ibid.

iv J. Katz, et al., "Seven- to 10-Year Outcome of Decompressive Surgery for Degenerative Lumbar Spinal Stenosis," *Spine* 21, no. 1 (1996), pp. 92–97.

IT STILL HURTS! WHAT DO I DO?

The hard truth is that some back pain is impossible to diagnose, resistant to treatment, and incredibly frustrating to both patient and doctor. The point of *I've Got Your Back* isn't to provide definitive answers to back pain questions—those answers don't exist—but to help the patient understand when surgery may and may not help.

I know, though, that it's maddening to try option after option and have none of them work. That's why spinal surgery gets done so often in the face of less-than-promising odds; when you feel like you've tried everything, even risky procedures start sounding tempting.

My advice to those patients is: patience. There is *always* something else to try.

Pain management is a burgeoning field, and physiatrists are making progress in helping patients handle discomfort that might otherwise drive them to a surgeon. Although some pain medications are being reevaluated in light of dangerous side effects, there are still many safe alternatives. Back pain—and chronic pain in general—also often responds well to some of the alternative treatments mentioned in section III. Some of those treatments, like acupuncture and herbs, are somewhat outside the realm of medicine, but it can't hurt to try them—something you can't say of surgery.

So try physical therapy, or a chiropractor. Get one of the books on back pain, and try its suggestions. Get more exercise.

Even for patients with the most resistant back pain, the outlook isn't necessarily grim. For many patients, the pain often decreases or even disappears, for reasons we don't understand any better than we understand the reasons for the pain in the first place. Patience is one of the best weapons we have in the fight against back pain.